Outlining Tinnitus

A comprehensive guide to help you
break free of the ringing in your ears

Mark Knoblauch PhD

Kiremma Press
Houston, TX

Printed in the United States of America

Disclaimer: This book is not intended as a substitute for the medical advice of licensed medical professionals. The reader should regularly consult his or her physician in any matter relating to his/her health and particularly with respect to any symptoms that may require diagnosis of a medical attention.

www.authorMK.com

ISBN: 978-1-7320674-2-4

This book is dedicated to all individuals who have to deal with the frustration, annoyance, and often debilitating effects of tinnitus.

TABLE OF CONTENTS

Introduction

If you have purchased this book, it's likely that you or someone close to you has been living with the annoying effects of tinnitus. Whether it be a high-pitched hiss or a low, pulsating howl, tinnitus can be annoying if not debilitating. The unending sound invades all aspects of your life, from your sleep to your most intimate moments. Particularly frustrating is that no one else can detect what you are experiencing. This often leaves those around you empathetic yet not quite fully understanding the frustration you are experiencing. And because most types of tinnitus are subjective in nature, there are no medical tests that can verify its presence other than a description provided by you the patient, along with an array of notable psychological characteristics such as irritability, agitation, or anxiety.

I am familiar with all of these aspects, as I too have dealt with constant tinnitus for over 15 years now. And as a sufferer, I can attest that my initial dealings with tinnitus were not pleasant. But after many years of living with tinnitus as well as other conditions of the ear, my tinnitus is now an afterthought even though it has not diminished over time. To be clear, my tinnitus is an afterthought as long as I'm not directly focusing on my ear directly, anyway. If during the day I choose to mentally check in to see if my tinnitus is still there, I find that it is *always* there. However, if I ignore it and stay focused on whatever else I'm doing, I never notice my tinnitus. Similarly, avoiding situations where I have to sit in seemingly dead silence – such as being alone in an unusually quiet room – also helps me avoid reminders of my tinnitus. Other times, having access to background noise such as a ceiling fan, soft music, or conversation can all serve as excellent methods for suppressing the constant hissing sound that is sitting there patiently, waiting to push through my subconscious thought process and remind me of its presence.

Despite its relatively common occurrence, tinnitus is a strangely evasive condition that has puzzled scientists and doctors for decades. Medicine and science have learned a lot about the ear, and we have pinpointed the cause of many conditions of the inner ear, including some which are much less common than tinnitus. However, we haven't progressed as far as we might hope when it comes to tinnitus. Some of the difficulty in targeting a final cause of tinnitus appears to lie in the fact that it may be more complex than we think, and as such may not be the result of a single issue but rather a complex mix of events that emerge as a single condition. Much like the common cold, the seemingly minor events associated with tinnitus have proven to be quite difficult in solving, thereby pushing a cure for tinnitus further down the road than was likely suspected.

Despite the fact that a cure eludes us, many tinnitus patients have had treatment success with suppressing the symptoms of their tinnitus to the point that it no longer affects them. Tinnitus that may have once been extremely frustrating and annoying has become effectively non-existent. Whereas this progression occurred for my own tinnitus, I want to be able to share my success with you and anyone else suffering from tinnitus. That in effect is the essence of this book – to help you manage the effects of tinnitus and either get back to or maintain your way of life in a way that tinnitus is nothing but an afterthought to you as well.

Therefore, this book is outlined to not only provide you tips and techniques to help you deal with your tinnitus, but it is also designed to serve as a resource to help you learn more about this frustrating condition. We will start off by reviewing the relevant anatomy of the inner ear, highlighting those areas suspected to be involved in tinnitus. Next we'll review the most relevant and recent research into tinnitus, including the variety of suspected causes. By understanding the research associated with tinnitus, it can help you have a better understanding of just how complex tinnitus is and also help you understand how difficult it can be to establish the source of your tinnitus.

Because I have had a long history with tinnitus myself, I'll next outline for you my own experience with tinnitus – from when I first noticed it while sitting on a couch one day to now having to hear it hissing incessantly in both ears. We'll then look at treatments associated with tinnitus, both in terms of those treatments that have been put through the rigors of science as well as a few of the unproven yet reportedly beneficial treatments that are available. Next we'll explore a few of the medical conditions that are often associated with tinnitus, followed by a look at how tinnitus affects a patient's quality of life, focusing on not only the reported effects of tinnitus but also taking a look at the financial burden that can result. I have also added a chapter dedicated to those individuals who provide care for a tinnitus patient, as well as a discussion on how to help prevent tinnitus.

If you or someone you know has been newly diagnosed with or is living with tinnitus, this book has been written for you. You will likely have a series of initial frustrations in dealing with tinnitus just like I and so many other sufferers have encountered, and this book is written to help get you through those initial stages of tinnitus and work to help you manage your tinnitus over time. My hope is that this book will make you a better-informed tinnitus patient as well as one that will be able to maintain a normal lifestyle despite having the annoying ringing in your ears that may initially seem to be quite overbearing.

If you are a patient, rest assured that tinnitus is a very manageable symptom. As you will read in this book, the initial stages of dealing with chronic tinnitus are typically the worst, but over time you can expect that tinnitus becomes less and less noticeable. There are a wealth of treatment options to help diminish the perception of tinnitus, and matching your own tinnitus experience with the right treatments can make an amazing difference in your perception of tinnitus, with the hope of ultimately returning you to a quality of life that existed prior to your tinnitus. Now, let's take a journey together to get you on your path to being free from the frustrating grip of tinnitus.

Chapter 1: Anatomy of the Ear

TO UNDERSTAND TINNITUS, we have to first understand the structures suspected to be involved in causing tinnitus. You read that right – *suspected* to be involved. Unfortunately, despite a long and detailed history of investigation into just what tinnitus is, medicine has not yet figured out the precise set of events or structures responsible for triggering tinnitus. However, because of continued research, our understanding of tinnitus continues to improve over time, thereby leading us down the road to what we can hope to be an eventual cure.

Whereas research suggests that the inner ear plays a significant role in tinnitus we'll focus most of this chapter on the structures of the highly intricate ear. While you may think of your ear as that flap of cartilage on the outside of your head, most of the functional portions of the ear are located deep in the skull, behind your eardrum. Hidden within our temporal bone are complex structures responsible for the detection of sound, along with additional structures responsible for sensing motion that allows us to maintain body position and move around in our environment. Unfortunately, because the structures of the ear are so intricate, they are also quite delicate. This in turn makes the ear quite susceptible to damage such as can occur through physical trauma (e.g. punch to the head) or disease as well as through sound-based trauma such as might occur in response to long-term, loud noise. In order to understand how these factors contribute to tinnitus, we'll now take a detailed look at the structures involved in sound detection and interpretation.

Outer ear

Located mostly outside of the skull, the outer ear is the portion of the ear that we can see (Figure 1.1). This includes the large cartilage-based *pinna* along with the ear canal that forms within the temporal bone and leads to the eardrum. The function of the outer ear is to funnel sound to the eardrum, and as it is largely situated well away from the intricate middle ear and comprised of nothing more than skin, cartilage, and a tube formed through the outer temporal bone, the outer ear is not suspected to have involvement in tinnitus.

Middle ear

The middle ear is a cavity formed within the skull. It is the air-filled portion of the ear located behind the eardrum and housed completely within the temporal bone (Figure 1.1). This portion of the ear

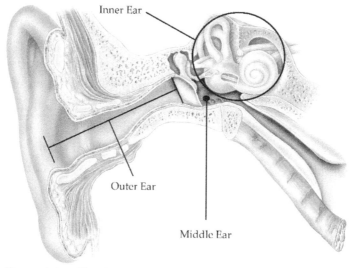

Figure 1.1. The three sections of the ear include the outer ear, middle ear, and inner ear. Issues involved with tinnitus are located within the labyrinth portion of the inner ear.

contains the three small bones – the malleus, stapes, and incus – that transfer sound from the eardrum to the inner ear. With the exception of one medical condition that we will discuss (otosclerosis), the middle ear is not thought to be involved specifically with tinnitus.

Inner ear

The inner ear is the portion of the ear responsible for both conversion of sound waves to neural impulses and also for the perception and interpretation of the head's position. The inner ear is comprised of highly sensitive structures which in turn make the inner ear susceptible to injury. Because of the high level of involvement of the inner ear specific to sound and movement detection, the inner ear is one of the most intensively studied areas of vertebrate anatomy and physiology[1]. Despite its small size, damage to the intricate components of the inner ear can affect hearing as well as equilibrium, and even minor disruptive events can trigger several symptoms such as motion sickness, vertigo or nausea.

There are two predominant structures that comprise the inner ear – the cochlea and the vestibular system (Figure 1.2). Together, these two structures make up what is known as the *labyrinth*. It should be noted that the labyrinth organs are not free-standing organs; rather, they are actually tunnels that exist within the temporal bone. These tunnels contain membranes that serve to contain the fluid (i.e.

'endolymph') housed within the labyrinth. Tinnitus is largely thought to be localized to the auditory

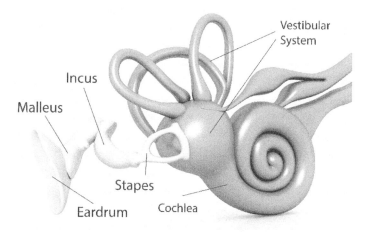

Figure 1.2. Sound detected by the eardrum is transmitted through the ear bones (malleus, incus, and stapes) to the fluid-filled cochlea, where nerve cells send the sound signal to the brain

portion of the labyrinth, and so for the purposes of this book we will not discuss the structures involved in the vestibular system.

Cochlea

The cochlea is an area of the inner ear that forms a 3-4cm long coiled, bony cavity resembling a snail shell within the temporal bone[2] (Figure 1.2).

Structurally, the cochlea is embedded within some of the most dense bone material in the body[3] (Figure 1.3). The main function of the cochlea is to convert sound waves from the eardrum into nerve impulses, which are then sent to the brain for interpretation as sound. This occurs as a result of

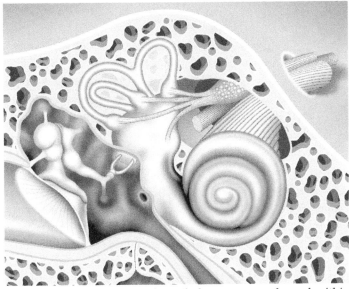

Figure 1.3. The cochlea and vestibular system are housed within the matrix of the temporal bone. Though actually formed by the bone, the labyrinth organs are lined with membranes that house the endolymph fluid of the inner ear.

vibrations received from the small bones of the middle ear, known collectively as the ossicles. As the eardrum moves in response to sound waves, it transmits vibrations to the ossicles. One of the ossicles, known as the stirrup, is attached directly to the thin oval window membrane located on the cochlea. As the stirrup moves, its attachment to the oval window membrane generates vibrations which are then transmitted into the fluid contained within the cochlea. It is the movement of this cochlear fluid that generates the stimulus that our brain interprets as sound.

Sound reception within the cochlea

Our sensation of hearing is really a coordinated event involving two different components. First, structures within our skull *detect* the sound and transmit it to the inner ear and eventually to our brain. Then, our brain *interprets* the sound which allows us to perceive and understand the source of the sound, which we may then recognize as a speech pattern, a baby crying, or perhaps an airplane flying overhead. Science has largely figured out how sound is detected within our ear specific to the structures involved and how they work for the detection of sound. However, our understanding of how the brain interprets sound is actually quite poor. We have established the areas of the brain that are involved in hearing, and we have figured out how signals are sent from the ear to the brain, but how the brain can interpret and process signals received by our ears remains relatively poorly understood.

What we do know is that processing of sound signals is much more complicated than once thought. That helps explain why a relatively common problem like tinnitus still remains unsolved both in terms of a cure but also specific to just what is causing it. Because of the complexity involved in the hearing process it is important that we first take a look at the procedures involved in sound interpretation since, as we will discuss later, there appears to be some degree of association between hearing and tinnitus.

Inside of the cochlea is a structure called the organ of Corti that snakes its way through the length of the cochlea. The organ of Corti contains approximately 15,000 hair cells responsible for detecting vibrations within the cochlear fluid, known also as endolymph[4]. Higher-pitched sounds cause vibrations or 'waves' within the endolymph that activate hair cells near the oval window, while lower-pitched sounds stimulate hair cells further down the length of the cochlea. The variation in the type of hair cells that are activated occurs because the hairs throughout the cochlea are of different lengths. Short, stiff hairs are near the oval window while longer, more 'flexible' hairs are found near the far end of the organ of Corti. This organization of the cochlea is how you are able to detect different frequencies of sound – shorter hair cells respond to higher-pitched sounds like those produced by a ringing bell, while lower-frequency sounds (such as a hum) stimulate the longer hairs near the end of the organ of Corti.

What all of this means is that varying sounds are detected along different areas of the organ of Corti within the ear. The brain's interpretation of these various sounds are what we understand as hearing (and interpretation) of sound. As mentioned previously, the structures involved in this process are highly intricate, and as a result are quite susceptible to damage. Consequently, damage to a specific part of the cochlea can affect an individual's perception of that corresponding sound frequency. For example, damage to the organ of Corti near the oval window, where higher-pitched sounds are detected, would likely reduce an individual's ability to hear sounds such as a bird chirping. Similarly, damage to the organ of Corti near its furthest end would decrease hearing of low frequencies, such as occurs with many aspects of normal speech.

Not all hearing loss is related to acute types of damage (i.e. trauma), though. As we age, our hearing can be expected to decrease over time in a process known as *presbycusis*. Most of this age-related hearing loss is attributed to slow-developing changes within the inner ear. No one single factor is associated with age-related hearing loss, but it is thought to result in part from degeneration of the cochlea over time[5].

Signal transfer to the brain

One of the fascinating features of the ear is that it has the ability to transfer sound vibrations into electrical signals, which your brain then interprets as sound. This process, though quite technical in its detail can be pared down to a few key steps that help outline how we hear normal sound, and may play an as yet undetermined role in tinnitus as well.

The tips of hair cells extend out into the middle of the fluid-filled cochlea in order to detect vibrations within the endolymph. When the right frequency of vibration within the endolymph stimulates a particular hair cell, it initiates a process that converts the fluid vibration into an electrical signal that is sent via nerves to the brain. This process is initiated as the wave of endolymph hits the appropriately "tuned" hair cell, which causes that hair cell to move slightly. So slightly, in fact, that it has been stated that the amount of motion actually occurring is equivalent to the top of the Eiffel tower bending about an inch[6]!

The small bit of movement of the hair cell causes tension to develop at the base of the hair cell. This then triggers the release of a chemical (i.e. "neurotransmitter") from special cells located at the base of the hair cell. This neurotransmitter is sensitive to detection by nerve cells, so as the neurotransmitter is released it thereby activates another nerve responsible for transmitting the signal to the brain. The brain then determines the frequency of the hair cell responsible for the detected signal and assembles the signal into what we interpret as sound.

Take a minute and think about the detail involved in the process of detection and interpretation of sound. Sit quietly and absorb all of the sounds around you. You will quickly realize just how much activity your ears are processing at every moment. Now think about how easily you can determine the frequency, loudness, and direction of each sound, including what are likely multiple sounds all at once. Or how your brain categorizes different sounds, and how it can separate out the noise from the important sounds. Or how you can recognize the distinct sound of a familiar voice out of 1,000 others. Now perhaps you can gain a better appreciation for the function of the ear and the duty of the brain in processing all of this information – constantly. Furthermore, think of how these sounds are being processed every moment that you are conscious, and how the majority of them are suppressed, interpreted by your brain as being unimportant. It is quite a fascinating system and one that people probably give little thought to until their hearing has been affected.

Summary

Although tinnitus is not fully understood, it is known that there is an association between tinnitus and the inner ear. This chapter was designed to provide an overview of the main areas and structures of the inner ear, which we will refer back to in the next chapter specific to the particular components of the ear.

As we have outlined, the structures of the inner ear are responsible for the detection of sound and are highly intricate in their design. Damage to any of the structures of the inner ear can have significant impact on our hearing, regardless of whether that damage is from physical trauma or acoustic-type trauma that may occur as the result of chronic exposure to loud noise. By detailing the structures of the ear, it provides us a foundation that can help us better understand the mechanisms involved in tinnitus and how certain treatments target specific areas of the ear.

Chapter 2: What is tinnitus?

IF YOU HAVE TINNITUS, you are certainly familiar with the effects of that frustrating 'sound' that seems to be resonating from either outside of your ear or within your head. Depending on your particular type of tinnitus, you may be perceiving a high-pitched ringing, a static-type sound, howling, or even clicking, but regardless of the type, it can be extremely annoying. Whereas in the previous chapter we looked at the intricate anatomy of the inner ear's auditory system, we'll now look into just what tinnitus is as well as what anatomical events are theorized to cause tinnitus.

A brief history of tinnitus

If there is any disease of the ear with a longer or more thorough history of documentation than tinnitus, you'd be hard-pressed to find it. Medicine has come a long way from the days of treating what was once described as a 'bewitched ear' by infusing a couple of oils into the ear[7], yet the frustrating symptom of tinnitus still survives yet today – almost as if tinnitus has become the veritable 'cockroach' of medicine.

Treatments for tinnitus-like conditions have been reported in various versions of medical literature for thousands of years. The earliest known is the aforementioned "bewitched ear" treatment described on the Ebers papyrus (written around 1550 BC) which includes a treatment that requires the mixing of balanities and Frankincense oils together before inserting the mixture into the external ear[7]. Whether this was specific to tinnitus itself or even effective as a treatment is not exactly known, as the information contained on the papyrus was interpreted using hieroglyphs (i.e. pictures). However, it does suggest that tinnitus may well have been treated as far back as the time of the ancient Egyptians.

Later, Mesopotamian texts thought to arise around 700 BC included over 20 different ear conditions related to tinnitus[7]. Treatments included consumables such as turmeric or putting mustard in beer, but also involved the specific use of chants for some described types of tinnitus[7]. Later, Hippocrates described how the buzzing in the ears stops if a sound is made[8], suggesting that masking of tinnitus can help reduce its severity. Celsus later (~30 AD) suggested exercise, rubbing, and gargling as possible treatments, along with dieting and the insertion of drugs into the external portion of the ear[9].

These reports indicate that tinnitus has been problematic enough to warrant medical treatment for thousands of years. Over time, the recorded treatments for tinnitus became somewhat more rational, such as the medieval age's use of a rod to induce a negative pressure on the eardrum[7], yet also presented a few relatively odd treatments that included drilling a hole into the skull to allow the tinnitus-generating wind to escape the head, or fastening hot loaves of bread to a tinnitus patient's ears to induce perspiration[7]. As the nineteenth century arrived, treatments for tinnitus fell more in line with what we may think of as 'modern medicine'. These treatments included electrical stimulation to suppress tinnitus, precise loud sounds, massage, and even the first attempts at surgery[7].

While the historical treatments used in battling tinnitus may sound a bit radical or even far-fetched, it is important to remember that medicine has taken a similar path over time. The very reason that we see these treatments as "odd" is because they have been proven ineffective over time, or in some cases the premise for the treatment has been shown to make no logical sense. Looking at the situation differently, if medicine had not advanced past the days of tying hot bread loaves to your ears, you can bet that we as humans would still be engaging in that practice. But through our improvement of medicine, brought about as a result of the scientific process (discussed in more detail in Chapter 5), prior medical techniques become obsolete and more beneficial treatments are utilized. While we're not 'there' yet in terms of a treatment that eliminates tinnitus, every unproven or discontinued treatment further narrows down our focus into treatments which show potential.

What is tinnitus

To understand tinnitus we have to take a look into what it is that we currently understand about the condition itself. As we have touched on in the previous section, our knowledge of tinnitus is improving, and although we don't know yet what exactly causes tinnitus, we are making valuable headway into understanding what *doesn't* cause tinnitus. This two-pronged approach helps ensure that we are moving forward in medicine to increase our understanding of just what is involved with this annoying and frustrating symptom.

Tinnitus is a word derived from the Latin *tinnire* ("to ring") and is defined as the perception of sound without a true external source[10]. In other words, a tinnitus patient feels as though they are hearing something even though nothing in the environment around them is generating that perceived 'sound'. Therefore, the sound patients feel that they are hearing is actually generated internally from some as-yet-undetermined source. This perceived sound can take on many different forms, including ringing, hissing, or buzzing, and can be both intermittent in nature as well as coming in repetitive bursts[11].

Depending on the tinnitus sufferer, the perceived source of tinnitus may be reported as either originating from within one ear (unilateral), both ears (bilateral), or from inside the head itself[11]. Furthermore, the overall degree of tinnitus can range from barely perceptible to extremely loud and/or distracting.

Although the perceived location as well as the overall loudness of tinnitus can differ for each individual, the type of tinnitus an individual experiences is typically grouped into a particular classification. One such grouping defines tinnitus as either *primary* or *secondary.* Primary tinnitus has no recognizable source such as an underlying injury or disease and may occur in association with hearing loss[12]. Without a specific source of the tinnitus, primary tinnitus has no known cure and the treatment regimen may consist of a variety of options including counseling, medication, or dietary changes[12]. Secondary tinnitus, on the other hand, is associated with a known, specific event such as an auditory disorder or disease. This type of tinnitus can be treated by focusing on the underlying condition causing the tinnitus, which may include something as simple as ear wax buildup but can also be caused by more involved conditions such as hypertension. By treating the primary condition, secondary tinnitus can often be positively affected as well.

Another categorization for tinnitus is to group it as either *subjective* or *objective* in nature[13]. Subjective tinnitus is the more common form and occurs when a patient reports a unique sound (e.g. hissing, ringing, etc.) when there is no true externally-detectable sound. Most types of tinnitus we are associated with fall into the subjective tinnitus category. Objective tinnitus occurs when there is an actual sound event near the ear that can be heard by a medical practitioner with the use of a stethoscope. Often, the source of objective tinnitus is actually the movement of blood flow around the ear[10].

Causes of tinnitus

Research into the events involving tinnitus has been intensely studied for decades. In fact, determining the specific factors involved in tinnitus has been called one of the most controversial issues in medicine[10]. While science has made great strides in narrowing down the basic mechanisms of tinnitus, the precise cause of tinnitus along with the entire scope of events that cause it remains elusive[14].

Tinnitus can be triggered by several factors. Prolonged exposure to noise is the most common cause, triggering up to 22% of cases[15]. Additional originating events for tinnitus can include head and/or neck injury (17%) and infection (10%), along with other medical conditions (13%) such as disorders affecting the central nervous system[15] (e.g. meningitis) or issues involving cerebral blood flow[16] (e.g. stroke). One's work environment can increase the risk for tinnitus as well. For example, among military veterans, tinnitus has been reported to be the most common service-related condition requiring disability compensation[17]. Psychological factors can also play a role, as tinnitus has been shown to occur in response to stress or other emotional factors[18].

Although tinnitus can occur on its own, it has also been reported in conjunction with other medical conditions of the ear. Ménière's disease, acoustical neuroma, and depression/anxiety[19] have all been reported to involve tinnitus in many cases. Similarly, orthopedic factors such as disorders of the temporomandibular (i.e. jaw) joint can trigger tinnitus[20]. We will discuss many of these associated conditions in a later chapter.

While the onset of tinnitus can have a variety of factors, the actual structural cause of tinnitus is not

31

as well understood. In the majority of cases, tinnitus seems to arise from issues within the cochlea[11, 16]. Particular issues can include lesions brought about by traumatic noise, age-related hearing loss, or pharmaceutical drugs that can be damaging to the structures of the ear[11]. Furthermore, physical changes within the ear, such as growth of a benign tumor on the auditory nerve can also trigger tinnitus[21]. In fact, it has been suggested that if precise enough technology is used, some degree of cochlear deficiency will be noted in individuals with tinnitus[22].

For some patients, though, tinnitus can begin without any specific event that the patient can identify[16]. In these patients without a known trigger that initiated their tinnitus, it has been theorized that over time an alteration to the components of the auditory system occurred which then generated the effects of tinnitus[11].

Why such events would trigger a phantom sound from the ear remains somewhat of a mystery. Initial beliefs were that tinnitus was localized to the ear[23]. This makes sense from a general view, as the symptoms associated with tinnitus are typically reported as a perceived 'sound' from the ear. However, over 75% of tinnitus cases are determined to originate from either the acoustic nerves or specific issues involving the central nervous system[24], indicating that tinnitus is not localized to just the structures of the ear.

Evidence looking at hearing loss in conjunction with tinnitus further suggests that tinnitus does not solely involve the ear. For example, patients exhibiting tinnitus often have normal hearing[23, 25, 26]. Similarly, people with hearing loss do not consistently report having tinnitus[27]. Hearing loss is *often* reported in conjunction with tinnitus, but not always. Furthermore, in people with both hearing loss and tinnitus there is no consistency between the degree of decreased hearing and the level or type of tinnitus the individual experiences. In other words, people with minimal hearing loss can have severe tinnitus while people with severe hearing loss may have very low levels of tinnitus.

Perhaps the most solid evidence indicating that tinnitus is not localized just to the ear is that even when the auditory nerve is cut, tinnitus can persist[28, 29]. Whereas the auditory nerve is responsible for sending signals from the cochlea to the brain, it would seem logical that severing this connection would cease any improper signaling such as that which might be caused by tinnitus. However, as tinnitus can persist even when this neural connection is cut, it lends strong evidence that tinnitus is due to more than ear damage alone[16].

Several brain structures have been noted as potentially being responsible for or at least involved in tinnitus. Those structures and the theoretical framework behind their involvement in tinnitus are beyond the scope of this book. Briefly, some of these structures include the thalamic auditory nucleus[16], the cerebral cortex[30], the olivocochlear bundle, and the inferior colliculus[16]. Focusing future research on these areas can help improve our understanding of the primary source of tinnitus and allow targeted therapies to be developed.

Epidemiology of tinnitus

Epidemiology is the study of the occurrence of a disease such as investigating how many people are affected, how they became affected, and what may predispose an individual to getting a disease. Because tinnitus has no real measurable characteristics other than subjective information (i.e. what the patient describes), it can be a bit difficult to get consistent, accurate data on the prevalence, or actual occurrence, of tinnitus. Consequently, much of what we know about tinnitus occurs through either physician reports or through the use of surveys in which respondents answer specific questions about tinnitus. Therefore, survey quality is important, and the information derived from patient surveys must be analyzed in proper context. For example, a survey asking if an individual hears a perceived sound in his or her ear is not necessarily indicative of tinnitus, and does not outline how long the sound has been present. Rather, the survey must be specific enough to make it clear that the noise is in fact true tinnitus. Only survey results which have been deemed scientifically reliable and valid after a careful analysis of the survey design should be used for tinnitus-related research.

Specific to the epidemiology of tinnitus, individuals suffering from the condition should know that they are not suffering alone. Tinnitus is often described as a very common condition. Using self-reported survey data, researchers have found that approximately one-fourth of individuals in the United States report feeling the effects of tinnitus, and almost 8% experience frequent tinnitus[31]. However, such results do not tell the whole story of the overall effects of tinnitus, as the actual prevalence may be much higher given that only about 1 in 10 individuals with persistent tinnitus seek medical attention[32]. Furthermore, because tinnitus has many unique forms and variants (i.e. type, severity, etc.), it can be challenging for researchers to establish a true prevalence[16].

The likelihood of an individual having tinnitus is known to increase as that individual ages. Adults in the 60 to 69 year age group have the highest occurrence of tinnitus, with almost 33% of this age group reporting tinnitus[31]. Some studies have shown that after this age tinnitus prevalence continues to increase, while other studies report that there is a decreased rate of tinnitus after age 70[15, 26]. Similarly, there is conflicting research as to whether tinnitus *severity* increases with age, as reports indicate both no effect of age on tinnitus severity[33] as well as a positive effect of age and severity[34].

Though tinnitus is often associated with older individuals, it has been reported that children have tinnitus at rates similar to adults[35]. For example, from 7-16% of young Americans report a whistle or beep in their ears[36], and 60% report temporary ringing of their ears after going out[37]. Similarly, tinnitus in children is reported to be at a level equal to that of adults[35], though it has been suggested that it can be somewhat difficult to estimate tinnitus prevalence in children[23]. Interestingly, it has been suggested that children have a decreased stress level in response to tinnitus as compared to adults[35].

Despite the common occurrence of tinnitus in their age group, children seem to be less apt to complain about tinnitus[38] and are less stressed by their tinnitus[35], possibly due to their belief that the tinnitus is normal[39] or a belief that any report of tinnitus may not be taken seriously[40]. However, as hearing loss is related to tinnitus, evidence that some young adults do alter their behaviors after hearing-based tests have occurred[41] is encouraging, particularly when research has shown that these same young adults are less concerned with hearing loss than other medical conditions[42].

Gender prevalence of tinnitus also appears to have inconsistent evidence. Some studies report a higher prevalence of tinnitus in males[43, 44] while others claim no difference between males and females[26].

Individuals with a body mass index greater than 30 (i.e. obese) have been suggested to be more likely to have tinnitus[43], but this has largely been discredited[45, 46]. Furthermore, those with pre-existing conditions including hypertension, diabetes, anxiety, or elevated blood lipids also experience tinnitus at a higher rate. In addition, individuals exposed to chronic loud noise (e.g. military) have a higher prevalence of tinnitus[31]. Interestingly, the overall prevalence of tinnitus is expected to continue to rise due to overall exposure to increasing professional and leisure noise levels[47].

Duration and severity of reported tinnitus

In terms of tinnitus, the term *duration* relates to the amount of time the patient has been inflicted with the condition. As we have noted for some patients, tinnitus is not always permanent and can even improve over time. One study reported that over 40% of patients had complete resolution of tinnitus after five years, and 57% had only mild symptoms[48]. Another study found that long-term tinnitus declined over time in up to 7% of tinnitus patients[49]. Other studies report less favorable long-term effects, including one study reporting that 80% of patients still have persistent tinnitus after five years[50]. Interestingly, when this same data is interpreted differently it indicates that 20% of patients *do not* report persistent tinnitus after five years. However, these reports of diminished tinnitus could be due to physical changes within the ear, or may simply be a result of the patient naturally 'getting used to' the tinnitus which can in turn improve one's tolerance of tinnitus[51]. Regardless, the data indicates that a significant portion of tinnitus patients may in fact be able to expect some level of relief.

'Severity' of tinnitus relates to the degree of impact tinnitus has upon an individual's quality of life. A patient reporting non-severe tinnitus would be classified as having a level of tinnitus that does not influence their self-reported quality of life. It is interesting to note that as we stated earlier, a significant portion (i.e. 90%) of individuals who have tinnitus do not seek medical treatment[32]. Therefore, it should be expected that for most people, tinnitus is quite tolerable. When tinnitus severity reaches a level that causes patients to have trouble coping with its effects, medical attention is typically sought[52]. And, if occurring in conjunction with another medical condition such as hearing loss or Ménière's disease, the added effects of tinnitus can cause further detriments to quality of life such as an increased stress level.

In conclusion

Tinnitus is a very intricate symptom that has been treated for thousands of years. As a symptom, tinnitus is not a specific medical condition itself but rather occurs as the result of some other underlying condition. Despite the relatively common nature of tinnitus, science remains unable to outline just what structures are involved in causing the phantom sound, though it is suggested that there is both an ear-specific component of tinnitus as well as a brain-specific factor that plays a role in the symptoms of tinnitus.

While medicine has made great strides in helping narrow down the most probable causes of tinnitus, there still remains much to be learned about just what tinnitus is, how it occurs, and how it can be effectively treated and/or eliminated. Much of what perplexes researchers and medical professionals is due to not only the wide range of tinnitus that can occur, but also the varying degrees and triggers associated with tinnitus as well as the type of patient that is affected by tinnitus. Furthermore, certain risk factors along with specific medical conditions can increase one's risk of developing tinnitus and may complicate treatment of the associated tinnitus.

As medicine continues to narrow down the anatomy involved in tinnitus, targeted treatments will be able to be developed that will likely cure or at least suppress significantly the often-debilitating effects of tinnitus. As we will discuss in Chapter 6, these future treatments can be pharmaceutical in nature or can be an improvement upon one of the several methods that rely on distracting the patient from tinnitus. However, until a clearer understanding of the underlying structures and causes involved in tinnitus can be outlined, a true cure remains elusive.

Chapter 3: Diagnosis

HEARING A PERCEIVED SOUND in your ear, without any actual outside source, it effectively the definition of tinnitus[15]. But just because you hear some sort of phantom sound does not mean that you are afflicted with incurable, "chronic" tinnitus. It may be that something as simple as a buildup of ear wax could be triggering your tinnitus[53], and a simple removal of the wax may therefore cease your tinnitus. Conversely, tinnitus can be triggered by a much more serious condition such as an acoustic neuroma that requires immediate attention.

The wide range of triggers associated with tinnitus highlights the fact that it is essential that you contact your medical provider upon noticing tinnitus in order that they can work with you to determine the degree and possibly the cause of your tinnitus. In receiving a prompt medical evaluation, any underlying condition can be addressed quickly. Or, if you are stricken with the relatively common tinnitus associated with age-related hearing loss, you can then begin a guided treatment protocol that will hopefully bring you some relief from the sound in your ears.

Remember that tinnitus itself is not a true medical condition, but is rather a symptom of a separate underlying condition[54]. Therefore, the *cause* of tinnitus (e.g. hearing loss, acoustic neuroma, etc.) will likely be your ultimate diagnosis, with the ever-present tinnitus being a related symptom. As such, upon contacting your doctor about your recently-discovered tinnitus you will probably be evaluated for several other medical conditions to determine the cause of the tinnitus (rather than simply confirming that you in fact have tinnitus).

To think of it another way, imagine going to your doctor for a runny nose and sneezing. Like tinnitus, both symptoms are quite noticeable and can cause you a good degree of annoyance. However, the chances are quite high that you won't leave the medical office with a diagnosis of a runny nose and sneezing. As both events are symptoms of another condition, your doctor will factor all of your symptoms together in order to come to a likely diagnosis such as a bout of allergies. Similarly, if you went to your doctor for pain in your shoulder, he or she will look for the underlying cause, which may be discovered to be a torn tendon. You may get medication to block the pain (i.e. the symptom that you are reporting), but the underlying condition must be dealt with in order to truly eliminate the pain.

Likewise, medical professionals view tinnitus as one symptom of an underlying condition. Their initial concern will likely be to ensure that you do not have the worst possible tinnitus-related conditions. As they eliminate the likelihood that the tinnitus is brought on by something serious, they will shift their focus towards less concerning causes for the tinnitus. For example, elevated blood pressure within the head[12], vestibular schwannoma (i.e. tumor), or narrowing of the carotid artery can trigger tinnitus[11], and in each case it is imperative that the underlying condition is treated rather than focusing just on the tinnitus. Furthermore, other ear conditions such as Ménière's disease, which can often be managed through lifestyle modifications such as diet, can cause tinnitus[55].

Tinnitus is somewhat unique in that not only is it a symptom of an underlying condition, but as a symptom it can also cause problems in and of itself. Much like pain, tinnitus can at times be more bothersome than its underlying cause. For example, tinnitus arising from the relatively common age-related hearing loss can trigger bouts of depression or anxiety, each of which can require medical intervention.

Despite its wide prevalence, there is no specific medical test used to verify the presence of tinnitus. Rather, during examination the medical professional will likely inquire as to the patient's medical history, with relevant factors including whether there is any hearing loss associated with the tinnitus, the patient's exposure to noise, current or recent use of medications, and whether there is any associated vertigo[12]. Along with a thorough medical history, the patient's description of any perceived sound in their ear is often the primary indicator of tinnitus[23].

In addition to a subjective evaluation, practitioners may inquire as to additional aspects such as outlining any additional effects that the tinnitus may have on the patient[11, 23]. To assist with this aspect, a variety of questionnaires are available that can be used to determine severity as well as specifics of the tinnitus such as outlining the location of tinnitus (i.e. in one ear or both), the length of time that the tinnitus has been present, and whether the tinnitus has any particular rhythm or pulse[12, 23]. These questionnaires include the Tinnitus Severity Index, the Tinnitus Handicap Inventory, the Tinnitus Reaction Questionnaire, and the Tinnitus Handicap Questionnaire[15]. Patients may also be asked questions relevant to any possible emotional or psychological issues[12], which can be both triggered by tinnitus or exacerbated should either condition be present prior to the diagnosis of tinnitus.

In most cases, the initial medical consultation and a determination of tinnitus severity – coupled with an ear examination and assessment of hearing – will be adequate to address the patient's tinnitus[11]. Certain indicators found during an initial exam such as a potential cause for the tinnitus or evidence of impairment from the tinnitus may warrant a more in-depth examination, and in some cases, such as tinnitus resulting from trauma or tinnitus accompanied by a sudden loss of hearing, immediate interaction may be required[11]. Furthermore, tinnitus that presents with a psychological condition such as severe depression or suicide must also be addressed immediately[11]. It has been estimated that approximately one-third of patients with tinnitus will need a referral for further care in order to evaluate for a variety of other underlying medical conditions[56].

In conclusion

Whereas tinnitus is a symptom, patients do not receive a true diagnosis of tinnitus in the same way that they don't receive a diagnosis of "pain". However, given the sometimes-severe nature of tinnitus, it is often treated similar to a medical condition in that it requires specialized treatment focused on reducing its severity. Upon evaluating a patient complaining of tinnitus, medical professionals will first focus on whether an underlying medical condition exists in order to treat that condition and potentially eliminate the tinnitus. Through a detailed medical history as well as the patient's description of the tinnitus, a treatment plan can be formulated that addresses the concerns (e.g. quality of life, anxiety, etc.) of the patient.

Chapter 4: My tinnitus story

IT WOULDN'T BE RELEVANT for me to write a book about dealing with tinnitus unless I offer my own experiences with high-pitched ringing in my ears. You read that right – ears. I have had noticeable tinnitus to some degree in both of my ears for almost fifteen years now. And, it has progressed from extremely distracting and frustrating in the beginning to effectively non-existent now. By outlining my own story, hopefully you can relate somewhat and see that there is hope on the horizon for dealing with your tinnitus.

Tinnitus was not the first ear-related issue that I experienced. In 2002, I took an accidental knee to the side of my head that triggered a condition known as *benign paroxysmal positional vertigo*, or "BPPV". Though quite frightening upon first encountering BPPV, it's actually a rather harmless condition that occurs when small crystals called *otoliths* are displaced within the equilibrium center of your inner ear. As my head reached a certain position – tilted back and to the right – the otoliths came into contact with nerves deep inside my inner ear that then caused signals to be sent that were interpreted by my brain as though I was physically moving. As a result, vertigo is typically experienced with BPPV, along with a bout of rapid eye movement known as nystagmus. Eventually I was able to get a final diagnosis which resulted in a relatively simple set of head maneuvers designed to reposition the crystals back to their proper location within my inner ear. Six months after my first symptoms of BPPV, and two days after my diagnosis, I was back to normal.

Fast-forward about three years. I remember clearly that first moment I recognized the presence of my tinnitus. I was sitting on a couch in my apartment when I noticed that my right ear was ringing quite loudly with a high-pitched tone similar to that feedback sound you often hear if two microphones were placed too close together. Now understand, I'd noticed short-term tinnitus before – after a monster truck show many years earlier, a few times after rock concerts, and after a few pheasant or dove hunting trips. But each time, the tinnitus had followed a distinctly loud event (e.g. rock concert, gunshot, etc.). Sitting on the couch that day, however, I could not rationalize any reason as to why my ear was ringing. At the same time, I wasn't too concerned about this new bout of tinnitus, either. Quite frankly, I assumed that it would be gone in a day.

That night, lying in bed, the sound was unbearable. The silence of the room amplified the hissing coming from my ear, forcing me to turn on my radio to a low volume in order to suppress the blaring of the tinnitus. I lied in bed, trying my best to figure out what could have caused this bout, realizing that there was simply nothing over the past few days that could have triggered this annoying sound. Eventually, I was able to distract myself with the combined sound of a ceiling fan along with the radio, and I eventually fell asleep.

The next day, the sound was noticeable immediately upon waking up. I don't know if it was actually louder or I just gave it more thought than I had previously. This got my mind racing, trying to figure out why it was there as well as how it got there. Consequently, the rest of the day was spent with me distracted, constantly performing mental 'checks' to see if the sound was gone. What I noticed was that if I was outside the tinnitus diminished somewhat, almost giving me a false sense of security that it was fading. But upon walking back indoors I found that the high-pitched hissing was still there, raging madly as if to firmly remind me of its presence.

And so the next few days went. The sound became overpowering if I thought about it, which occurred pretty much constantly. I noticed that when I gave my tinnitus a moment of my thoughts, the sound in my ear seemed to get louder. This made me try to avoid thinking about it, which in turn only made me think about it more as I kept forcing myself to find out if the sound was still there, seemingly holding on to some false hope that it would suddenly disappear. Yet every time that I performed my mental checks I found that it was still there. The tinnitus was *always* 'still there'.

Soon I realized that the sound in my right ear was not going away as it had so many times before when brought about by a loud event such as a gunshot. Eventually I began to accept the possibility that I was suffering the effects of long-term tinnitus. I knew what tinnitus was, and had even taught students about the effects of tinnitus in my classes. But, I blew off any initial concerns as I had always associated spontaneous long-term tinnitus with older age – and I hadn't yet reached my mid-30s. So, I sat back, and waited.

Despite my days and weeks of waiting, the tinnitus did not go away. As I slowly began to accept the possibility that I was in fact suffering from long-term tinnitus I also became more conscious of factors affecting my hearing. As such, I began to listen to a lower volume on my car stereo when driving. Similarly, I listened to the TV at a quieter volume. I plugged my ears during loud events like being at an athletic event as the crowd screams. This sudden shift in my mindset aligned with a growing acceptance that I may well be experiencing tinnitus for the long-term. This belief was evidenced by the fact that the ringing was still constant, overbearing, and annoying.

I had 'allowed' the noise in my ears up to this point – in terms of holding off any psychological or anxiety issues – only because I had the expectation that it wouldn't be lasting long and it would soon fade away. As the days wore on, my anxiety increased. I started to get nervous as bedtime approached, for I knew that I would have to hear that brutally loud ringing sound once I turned the TV off. And turning the TV off started a vicious cycle whereby I would hear the sound, which would in turn invade my mindset and increase my stress and anxiety, thereby keeping me awake longer, which made me notice the ringing in my ears more, and so on and forth. The sound in my ears was becoming unbearable.

Around this time of accepting that I was becoming a tinnitus sufferer, I began doing my research into tinnitus treatments. What I found was that there were a whole lot of so-called 'cures' and very few actual successful treatments. The problem was, the cures that I read about were typically found on those poorly-designed internet websites touting a miracle oil or pill. Reading deeper into those pages revealed that they were really nothing but shams. I had even noticed a couple of television commercials advertising tinnitus treatment that I had seen before but paid little attention to at the time. Now, I saw how they advertised their product designed to " . . . eliminate that annoying ringing in your ear", only to find that when doing a quick internet search that the reviews of the product were terrible.

As I shifted my investigation to the treatments backed by science, I found that there was at the time no true cure for tinnitus. There were a lot of *recommendations* such as to eliminate smoking (not an issue for me), reduce alcohol consumption (again, not an issue), avoiding being around loud noises (done), and reducing stress (which was only brought about by my tinnitus). There were also a lot of invasive (i.e. surgical) treatments that some claimed to be beneficial, but I wasn't convinced that my own tinnitus was at a level that I'd allow anyone to cut the side of my head open. Furthermore, the fact that the surgical options were *sometimes* successful wasn't convincing enough for me to even think of pursuing that option.

All possible causes of my tinnitus were investigated, including the possibility that it was just the result of impacted ear wax being pressed up against my eardrum. I didn't think ear wax was a viable concern, but given that the tinnitus was only in my right ear at the time I figured it could be a possibility. Therefore, I gave in and bought the "loosening" oil designed to loosen and eventually remove excess ear wax, but it had no effect. I even accepted one treatment option that suggested I could be having a form of 'swimmers ear' that results from residual water within the ear. That led me to buy some liquid drops that are designed to remove excess water from the ear canal. Again, to no avail.

As I tried these recommended treatments – albeit unsuccessfully – I noticed there was one consistently recommended treatment that involved a psychological aspect. With that treatment method, the intent was to form a sort of 'disassociation' with or suppression of the tinnitus, where you effectively avoid thinking about it. My initial thoughts were somewhat skeptical: *Sure, I'll just "ignore" this overbearing noise in my ear! After all, it doesn't dominate my sleeping patterns or constantly remind me of its presence or anything!*

Despite my initial dismissal of this treatment method, pushing aside my bias allowed me to absorb some of what the research was saying. As I read deeper into this treatment, it started to make a bit more sense. And, here's a quick example of how it works. Reading this book, you're likely sitting down, correct? Until reading this very sentence, did you notice the sensation of the chair under your rear end? How about the feeling of the shoes on your feet? The actual sensation was there as soon as you sat down or put your shoes on, but why did you quickly forget about the pressure on your butt or feet? The answer is that your brain suppressed the sensation in each area because 1) it was used to the sensation, 2) the sensation had no harm or danger associated with it, and 3) the sensation provided no meaningful information.

Think about it this way. You consciously sit down, and there is pressure on your butt from the weight of you sitting on the chair. Does your brain really need to concentrate on that sensation? Is there any potential for harm provided by that sensation? If you slip and fall and there is a sudden sharp pain from the wrist that you landed upon, that provides a key (and strong) sensation that your brain *needs* to focus on because it provides relevant sensations very important for your brain to focus upon. If you apply those same earlier questions, as sudden pain in your wrist after slipping is not something that your brain is used to, it *does* have harm or danger associated with it, and it *does* provide meaningful information. As such, your brain will effectively force you to focus on the sensation in your wrist, as it must be dealt with immediately.

The same does not hold true for tinnitus. Well, at first it may hold true, as it's a new sensation that does not have a real purpose in being there. But over time, you will find that it's 'just' tinnitus, and you have no need to focus on it. That is in effect the premise behind tinnitus behavioral therapy, and it is what I began to work on with my own tinnitus.

As I had mentioned earlier, there were times during the day that the tinnitus was much more noticeable than others. When outside, in a 'busy' room full of people, or when there was ambient noise such as other conversations or background noise, I never noticed the tinnitus at all. In fact I would flat out forget about it during those times. However, when going to sleep, sitting in a quiet room, or doing things like studying or riding in an elevator – or any situation where it's quiet and I wasn't distracted – the tinnitus had the potential to reach the 'unbearable' level.

So while I had been trying to avoid those situations which seemed to amplify my tinnitus, I also realized that I had been mentally focusing quite heavily on my tinnitus. I was constantly asking myself *"is it there?"*, which drew my consciousness over to the tinnitus and increased my anxiety upon realizing it was in fact still there. Truth be told, it had been there *every* time. I had to convince myself that it wasn't going anywhere, and that I in fact had tinnitus *for good*. And accepting that, I think, helped me tremendously in realizing that my tinnitus was there to stay and that there was no real reason to check in on it anymore.

As I started putting into practice this new mindset, I noticed that I started thinking about my tinnitus much less. In fact, I almost seemed to *welcome* my tinnitus as I found that even though it's there in my ear, it has no real effect on anything other than my own anxiety – if I let it get to me. By accepting that it is there, I began to be able to ignore it. Previously, I would consciously think about it with the hope that it was gone or diminishing, only to consistently find out that it was still there with a vengeance. By accepting my tinnitus, I actually began to think about it much less.

Over time, my tinnitus became nothing more than a passing thought. It was there all the time, but as I expected it to be there anyway, it had no real intrusion into my daily life. I would still involve an ambient sound at bedtime such as a fan or soft music, and I was still diligent in avoiding unnecessarily loud sounds such as in my car or at home, but otherwise I led a pretty normal life for the next few years despite the relatively loud hissing.

A few years later I started having some new issues in my right ear – the same ear as both the tinnitus and the earlier bout of BPPV. Gradually I noticed that there was a persistent 'howling' sound, similar to a constant wind blowing through a tube of sorts. And, I noticed that certain 'sharp' sounds, such as might occur with a hammer hitting a board, became painfully loud. This went on for a couple of years, even leading me to eventually seek guidance from an audiologist. Nothing was found, but it became extremely annoying as at times the howling sound diminished my hearing tremendously.

Furthermore, the howling became intermixed with a fluctuating pressure in my ear that some days almost rendered me deaf in the ear while at other times seemed non-existent. Throughout the occurrence of these new issues in my ear, though, the tinnitus never let up.

Around this same time I noticed that there was a small but persistent bit of tinnitus noticeable in my left ear. At first, this caused quite a bit of anxiety for me. With everything that was going on in my right ear, my left ear had been a sort of 'sanctuary' that provided me my best sound perception and was what allowed me to hear effectively. Now, with tinnitus showing up in my left ear also, I feared that the new complications (e.g. pressure, etc.) going on in my right ear would also show up in my left, effectively making me unable to hear clearly. Not deaf, necessarily, but rather unable to clearly hold a conversation without either using the word "*what?*" several times or requiring an exorbitant amount of concentration. When the howling in my right ear was bad I often had to resort to what I called "keyword conversations" in which I had to try to connect with specific words (i.e. keywords) in the other person's conversation in order to piece together what they were saying. If both ears became affected with a detrimental bout of howling, pressure, and tinnitus, I would have no real ability to hold a conversation in anything but the most silent of situations. As I said, this became a major source of anxiety for me at the time.

Eventually, the issues in my right ear led to random, violent bouts of vertigo. After almost three years of unanswered questions I was eventually diagnosed with Ménière's disease, a relatively obscure condition of the inner ear that triggers constant imbalance, vertigo, and pressure within the ear. My diagnosis with Ménière's led to an eventual treatment that was very successful for me and required a closely-monitored low-sodium diet. By reducing my daily sodium intake to no more than 1000 milligrams, the vertigo as well as the fullness and howling sounds in my ear eventually stopped. However, the tinnitus persisted.

Now, having had BPPV, tinnitus, and Ménière's, I can say without a doubt that tinnitus was the least problematic of the three conditions. By far. Tinnitus is always present, but has no real effect on my daily life – unless I let it. By contrast, BPPV and Ménière's (and actually Ménière's to a much, much greater degree) exerted significant impact on daily life as they involved bouts of vertigo. Tinnitus, by comparison, was to me nothing more than an annoyance, and so became even more irrelevant when dealing with Ménière's. Kind of the same way that someone might not worry about a leaky faucet when the bank is threatening to foreclose on the house.

Even though I no longer have issues with Ménière's or BPPV, I pay no attention to the tinnitus that I have. Currently, my tinnitus is more prevalent in my left ear, sounding as though it is coming from an area behind my left eyeball. As I mentioned earlier, it sounds relatively similar to that noise you hear when two microphones are in too close of proximity to each other. Not as ear-piercingly loud as that sound actually makes, by any means, but present nonetheless. When comparing a similar sound online, my tinnitus matches that which falls in the range of around 11,000-11,500Hz.

I still occasionally check in on my tinnitus or notice it at certain times, but it earns nothing more than the equivalent of a passing glance. By addressing and accepting that I have tinnitus, I have in turn been able to forget about it over time. It has been relegated to nothing more than the attention that I may give to a sore shoulder that I feel with certain motions. Despite a constant presence and no sign of it going away, I feel that I have won my battle with tinnitus. While I was once in a daily struggle that was clearly in tinnitus' favor, I now consider myself tinnitus-free given the infrequency with which I am affected by this condition. By retraining my thought process toward accepting my tinnitus, I have been able to suppress it to a level that allows me to now forget that it's even there.

As we'll discuss in the next chapter, the therapy that worked effectively for me is just one of the many treatment options available to help you overpower your tinnitus. With a vast array of tinnitus treatment options, even if one is not effective you can try another, and another, until you find the treatment option that works best for you. Over time, with treatment you will also likely notice that your tinnitus becomes less and less bothersome, to the point that you can also expect to pay no real mind to what once seemed an overbearing sound in your ear.

Chapter 5: Tinnitus Treatment

A FIRST REACTION THAT SOMEONE may have upon experiencing tinnitus is to simply search the internet for help and begin the treatment(s) outlined on some web page. While this is quite convenient in our digital age, it is not recommended. Although tinnitus typically has no established underlying cause, there are several medical conditions we have discussed that can trigger tinnitus. It is essential that as a sufferer of tinnitus you first receive a thorough medical evaluation to ensure that there is no treatable condition that is actually triggering your tinnitus. Once the primary cause for your tinnitus has been determined, it is important that you work with your medical provider to establish a treatment plan in order to find the best available options for your tinnitus.

A second reason to avoid the 'internet' style of treatment is that tinnitus is unique to each person. As we have discussed, there are several types of tinnitus out there that can occur in varying levels of severity. It is important as a patient that any treatment plan used is tailored to you alone. This could mean a special diet, behavior therapy, sound therapy, pharmacologic therapies, or even hearing aids. You must not fall into the trap of believing everything that you read on the internet when it comes to tinnitus. While there are some legitimate options available online, there are also a wealth of fraudulent offers and sham treatments, and it is important that you as a patient be able to understand how to separate the good information from the bad. Therefore, in the next section we're going to deviate a bit from tinnitus and look at what is known as the scientific method. By doing so, it will help you as a patient and a consumer better understand and separate those tinnitus treatments that have been proven to work versus what may work versus what *will not* work. This information can help prevent you from being taken advantage of as a tinnitus sufferer and also allow you to focus your treatment on the most viable options available.

The scientific process

Science is all about observations. If a researcher designs an experiment, he or she already has a predicted outcome. By observing what happens during the experiment, his or her prediction is supported or rejected. In some cases, predictions are relatively simple, such as *if I flip a coin, it will reveal 'heads' 50% of the time*. There is pretty much a one-in-two chance that the coin will show 'heads', as there are only two sides to the coin. If you drop the coin enough times, it's likely that you will find that there is an equal chance that heads or tails will occur 50% of the time. So, if you write down every outcome of your coin flips it should be an expected result that heads has just as much chance as tails in occurring.

Although that is a relatively simple example, in science it is never permitted to simply "assume". You still have to test your prediction, or *hypothesis.* There may be some unknown, small factor that influences your experiment. What if, for example, someone handed you a pair of dice that when rolled, came up as a "three" and "four" 84% of the time? Wouldn't that seem a little odd versus what you would predict? If so, your hypothesis would be refuted. A little further investigation may reveal that the dice were rigged to come up as a total of "7". So even though you expected that a random pair of dice would provide random pairs of numbers, you still have to test your prediction to ensure that there is not some unknown factor influencing the results.

As I mentioned, making predictions using coins or dice are quite simple examples. Things get much more complicated in terms of experiments and predictions when it comes to fields like medicine or psychology. If a researcher designs a drug with the intent for that drug to cure a specific condition, it is relatively simple in concept to design the drug molecule to fit and bind to a specific receptor in the body that should generate an action that the researcher intends. However, it is much more complicated to get that drug molecule to the area of the body it needs to be, or survive the digestive system, or stay in an active form long enough for it to perform its function. Furthermore, researchers also have to be able to predict any side-effects or unwanted conditions that may result from that drug. And, they have to show that whatever non-harmful effects occur do in fact occur consistently across several individuals with that condition. It can be a frustrating and difficult process, but it is essential for establishing the 'truth' about a product.

Unfortunately, establishing all of these factors takes both time and money. A researcher typically has to obtain a grant to pay to have the facilities, staff, and equipment to design their treatment (i.e. drug, tool, etc.). Furthermore, the researcher has to get approval to test their treatment by showing that what they are doing is both ethical and necessary – which can in itself be a long, drawn-out process. And if they reveal legitimate results – sometimes only in a test tube – they have to be able to show that their results can be replicated (i.e. repeated) across a wide variety of individuals. Once that occurs and there is a clear benefit, the researcher will most likely be able to start marketing his or her product. When done properly, this process can take years.

In light of the effort required to develop and test a potential treatment effectively, many people or companies have decided that it's much simpler to just forego all of the bureaucratic 'nonsense' and post some treatment online that they believe is effective. The problem in doing so is that there lacks real evidence that the treatment actually works. And, the person selling the treatment often knows that the product has no proof – especially when there is a potential financial gain in store for them if they can just convince enough people to buy the product.

Testing on subjects

In order to outline why it is important that products work across groups of people rather than just a single person, we need to look at what is commonly referred to as a *subject*, or an individual involved in experimental testing.

Humans are very similar but very different from each other. Stand two individuals of the same gender, height, and weight, next to each other and you might say that they are very similar. But, if you investigate deeper into what you can't see, you might find that one is allergic to a substance, or has high blood pressure, or maybe has an autoimmune disorder. In other words, looking at their outward appearance tells you nothing about particular details that you can't see, such as a medical condition. So, what may work or be safe for one of them might not be the case for both. This is a very simple example of how medical treatments work, and what works for one person may not work for all. However, if a researcher can show that a treatment works for *many* – even though it may not work for everyone – it can be cause for getting that treatment on the market.

In medicine, when something applies to a single entity, such as a person, location, or event, it is referred to as a *case.* For example, a flu outbreak at a school after a student returns from another country would be specific to that school, and is not particularly relevant to *all* schools. Therefore, that particular flu outbreak could be considered a case for that school. Similarly, if a patient is allergic to, say bacon, that would make his or her situation a case specific to him or her rather than an expected reaction for everyone as the vast majority of people are not allergic to bacon. Medical treatments apply similarly – if something works for one single patient, it doesn't necessarily mean that it is an effective treatment. However, if a treatment works for many people in a variety of situations (i.e. a "pool" of individuals), it is much more likely that the treatment truly works.

When it comes to tinnitus cures, there is no shortage of unique medical treatments available online. Many of these treatments have not only failed to go through the experimental design process as described earlier, but you will also find little evidence of consistent effects. Product descriptions may highlight a testimonial or two, but the question you as the patient and consumer have to ask yourself is whether that testimonial is valid and whether that single positive comment is worth you purchasing the product.

To outline how a useless product can seem to be a miracle cure, we can look at the tactics employed by shady sales people. There is an old phone scam that perfectly outlines how people can fall for false promises. Say you are a swindler and you are needing some cash. You call 40 people, 20 to whom you tout a new, 'hot' stock "A" and 20 to whom you tout stock "B". Stock A ends up doing poorly, so you never call back that group. But stock "B" does well, so you call back those people and say "see, I *told* you it would do well!". Knowing that your potential victims aren't quite sold on your service, you then tell half of the remaining people to buy stock "C", and half to buy stock "D". But only stock "D" ends up doing well. Therefore, you quickly call back the people in Group D, bragging about your skills as a stock genius and asking if they are finally ready to invest. Given what appeared to be your two hot recommendations, many in the group hand over money to you to invest for them. What the people in that group don't know is that 30 of your 40 original phone calls went unreturned due to a lack of performance. Consequently, they are quick to hand you their money to invest – after which you skip town, never to be seen again.

Internet-based tinnitus treatment options can work similarly. Sure, a person can tout the effects of a treatment, but how many did the treatment *not* work well for? If a $10 treatment works on 20 people but does not work on 80, is that a financial risk? Not really, and depending on the potential harm (hopefully there is none) it may be worth trying if nothing else has worked. But, what if that rarely successful treatment is a series of steps that take a month to complete, costs $400, and has the same success rate? You might be a bit hesitant to partake in such a treatment, and you rightly should be skeptical.

Some of the best validations you can find are independent clinical studies which involve the product's manufacturer shipping off their product for independent testing. But, putting a product through the testing phase costs money, and it is often much easier to just market the product to desperate people and convince them that it works. Maybe even pay the consumers to write a favorable review which will most likely make it onto the manufacturer's website. As potential customers look through the website, a bunch of favorable testimonials makes it tempting to purchase the product. But, isn't that really what effective marketing is supposed to do – convince you to buy a product? As the price you are willing to pay increases, you as the consumer and patient have to carefully decide if the product is worth the risk.

True effects vs coincidence

Along the same lines of establishing whether a product works on a single patient or is effective across a range of patients, it is also important to evaluate the facts about the treatment's reported effects. For example, say a person goes to a rock concert full of loud, booming speakers, and that night has a good bit of ringing in his ear. A friend gives him an oil to put in his ear, and when he wakes up, the tinnitus is greatly diminished. The second day after the truck rally, the ringing is gone. Does that mean that the oil fixed his tinnitus? Could it be that he didn't have the same chronic tinnitus that we all have, and therefore it went away on its own?

Given the circumstances, it's highly likely that the monster truck show caused temporary tinnitus – and therefore the oil had no real effect at all; rather, it was really just pure coincidence that the application of the oil coincided with the expected reduction in tinnitus. However, what do you suspect will happen when a few years later that same person runs into a colleague who is complaining of constant ringing in her ear for the past six weeks? Without a doubt, he'll be touting the effects of the oil. And given the long-term status of her tinnitus, she'll probably want to give it a try.

This scenario outlines the classic situation where either a misinterpretation or outright misinformation leads to belief in a treatment that doesn't work. Unfortunately, with chronic conditions that lead to desperate patients, there are individuals that capitalize on this desperation in order to sell treatments that have no realistic chance of working. I often see it myself online, and that is the main reason for my adding this 'introduction to research' to the chapter – to make you as a patient and consumer more aware. So, let's look a little deeper into what you should be assessing when it comes to a tinnitus treatment.

When science looks for a new treatment, it applies the treatment to one group (the experimental group) and no treatment to another identical group (the control group). Then, differences are evaluated between the groups, with the experimental group most likely expected to have a favorable outcome. For example, if there was a belief that low iron intake caused tinnitus, it could be *tested* by designing an experiment. The two groups would be equally comprised of individuals of similar gender and age as well as both duration and severity of tinnitus. In other words, you wouldn't want to apply the new treatment to a group of, say, females, and then use all males in the control group. Rather, you want consistency between groups. Therefore, you would establish each group so that they consist of similar individuals (e.g. tinnitus duration, gender, age, etc.). Then, for the experiment you would add the iron supplements to a meal for the experimental group while supplying the same meal to the control group, but without the added iron supplement. As long as everything else stays the same, any results occurring in the experimental group (such as an improvement in tinnitus after consuming additional iron) should be expected to be due to the treatment, and not random coincidence. If there is no improvement in the experimental group after the additional iron intake, it should be determined that the treatment has no effect.

The makeup of the experiment and control group is important as well. If, as mentioned, the groups are not made of similar individuals, you would effectively be comparing apples and oranges. For example, if you had one group that reported having tinnitus for six months and another group had tinnitus for at least ten years, keeping them separated in individual experimental and control groups would result in a major design flaw. However, if you *mixed* the groups so that some people with short-term and others with long-term tinnitus were in the same group, that would be acceptable as it creates a "pool' of evidence for the treatment.

It is also strongly recommended that the groups are comprised of enough people to capture all possible conditions that could affect the results. Do the groups capture all types of tinnitus, or just a specific one or two types? Is the long-term group all taking a certain medication, or have had a certain procedure? If so, these particular situations become *confounders* if they can influence the results. Say, for example, that ¾ of the people in the aforementioned experimental group were taking a tinnitus supplement that interfered with iron metabolism. If those same people then took the iron supplement, it would have no chance to get into the body and affect the tinnitus. Therefore, the experiment's results may end up showing that some people in the experimental group had an improvement in their tinnitus. However, if those same people were unknowingly the ones that were not taking the tinnitus supplement, it would make it look as though the experiment was not effective when really the iron was being prevented from working in some people. Therefore, it is important that the group's subjects are properly selected when designing an experiment.

Failure to explain the details of an experiment can become a problem for the researcher unless the particular patient details are made very clear, as the results of the study may only prove that the treatment is successful on a particular type of tinnitus, or in conjunction with another treatment, or *whatever the subject pool was comprised of.* Remember – assuming is not permittable in science. If a treatment has not been tested on a particular type of tinnitus (or patient), it cannot be assumed that the treatment will work until that factor is addressed in a scientific study.

What is all of this saying? Simple – it is recommended that you look for tinnitus treatments which have gone through the rigor of scientific testing if you're going to spend money on the treatment. There is actually much, much more that we could discuss regarding the scientific process, as we have just skimmed the surface. But, what we have discussed should help you to ask questions and read with more detail the evidence behind treatments that you encounter.

If there is no clear evidence or indication of a treatment's proof, I strongly suggest that you look elsewhere. At the same time, I am cognizant that there is no cure for tinnitus and as such, the cure remains 'out there' somewhere. If you look at how far we've progressed from the historical treatments used by the Mesopotamians, it's clear that we have made significant progress. And as we continue to eliminate ineffective treatments, we strengthen the pool of effective options while also expanding our search into new areas. When considering an alternative treatment for your own tinnitus, consider the risk as well as the evidence that exists for the treatment. The degree of proof that is required to use a particular treatment is ultimately left up to you.

Treatments for tinnitus

Now that you better understand how to wade through the available evidence regarding tinnitus treatments, we can begin to take a look at the more traditional treatments that are often used to battle tinnitus. We'll look first at the treatments most commonly used by medical professionals, and then also take a look at some of the less-proven treatments that you may find on the internet. Remember, treatment success is different from person to person when it comes to tinnitus. Therefore, if you do not respond to one treatment, it is essential that you do not give up – move on to the next and keep trying. The ultimate outcome is to improve your situation, particularly in your quality of life.

One of the major problems in treating tinnitus is that medicine still does not know exactly what causes tinnitus[57]. Consequently, specific treatments cannot be designed which target the true cause of the tinnitus. Furthermore, because several triggers of tinnitus exist as well as multiple types of tinnitus, it is not expected that one type of treatment would benefit all tinnitus patients. Still, medical advances are working to outline the most effective treatments, and when combined with the understanding that we are getting closer to answering the question of just what causes tinnitus, it should give hope to all tinnitus sufferers that relief may be coming soon.

In the following section we'll outline the various treatment options available for the treatment of tinnitus. First, we'll focus on those treatment options that have been put through the rigors of scientific review and then later examine a few of the non-traditional treatments. Typically, you will find that treatment for tinnitus generally falls into some form of pharmacological, psychological, or sound-based therapy, with varying degrees of success reported for each. Remember, as the cause of tinnitus can vary from person to person, there is no one treatment that is expected to work for everyone. Discuss the available options with your medical provider and work with him or her to develop a plan that can help provide you relief.

Pharmacologic treatment for tinnitus

The use of medication to reduce or eliminate tinnitus has been used for thousands of years[7]. In the past few decades, specific investigation has been done on a variety of drugs, and there have been relatively unflattering results. Part of this may lie in the fact that drugs typically target one specific protein (called a *receptor),* and given that many different tissues appear to be involved in tinnitus it can be difficult to find the right mix or type of medications. With this understanding, it is important to note that there is no current Food and Drug Administration (FDA) approved drug on the market that specifically targets the source of tinnitus[24]. Rather, many of the current pharmacologic treatment strategies for tinnitus do not necessarily focus specifically on eliminating the tinnitus but rather work to address associated conditions such as depression, anxiety, etc. For the purposes of this book, we will limit our discussion of pharmaceuticals to those drugs which have been studied to determine their direct effect on tinnitus, rather than on certain other conditions associated with tinnitus.

Interestingly, one of the most successful medications – intravenous lidocaine – was found to reduce tinnitus in 70% of patients[58]. However, the drug's effect was relatively short-lived, thereby requiring repeated administrations of the drug[10]. Unfortunately, the side effects associated with intravenous delivery of lidocaine outweighed the short-lived improvement in tinnitus, and its use as a therapy was discontinued[59]. Equally frustrating was evidence showing that oral delivery of lidocaine did not have as promising of results[60].

Betahistine is an anti-vertigo drug used to improve blood flow within the cochlea. Other medical conditions that involve the inner ear, such as

Ménière's disease, show positive responses to betahistine. However, tinnitus does not appear to respond favorably to betahistine treatment[61].

Intratympanic (i.e. 'through the eardrum') steroid injection has been shown to improve symptoms for certain inner-ear disorders such as Ménière's disease. However, intratympanic injection of dexamethasone as well as methylprednisolone have shown no benefit for reducing tinnitus based on subjective reports provided by patients[12]. Similarly, intratympanic injection of lidocaine has not been found to be beneficial as a treatment for tinnitus[62] despite the aforementioned favorable results when injected intravenously.

Antidepressant-type drugs have also been looked at for treating the direct effects of tinnitus. In most cases, reports indicate that there is no effect from antidepressant drugs; however, one study found that the antidepressant amitriptyline did decrease tinnitus severity in 95% of the experimental group, with only minor side effects including mild sedation along with dry mouth[63]. Another particular antidepressant – nortriptyline – showed a small effect on decreasing the loudness of tinnitus[64]. However, this particular study evaluated the drug in patients with both depression and tinnitus. Therefore, as we discussed early in this chapter, the results do not suggest that non-depressed patients should also expect a decrease in tinnitus loudness when taking nortriptyline. Unfortunately, antidepressants are also notorious for *causing* relatively short-term tinnitus[60]. Once stopping the drug, tinnitus typically resolves within a week; however, reports of up to seven months of continuous tinnitus have been reported following the use of amitriptyline[65].

Anti-anxiety drugs have also been investigated for their ability to directly improve tinnitus. One study showed that alprazolam use decreased tinnitus loudness in 75% of the experimental group[66], while another more recent study reported no improvement in tinnitus after taking a higher dose of alprazolam[67]. Clonazepam has also been shown to have a favorable effect on tinnitus-related factors including annoyance, loudness, and duration; however, almost half of the study participants taking clonazepam reported side effects that included drowsiness[68].

Anticonvulsant drugs have been shown to impact a very small component of tinnitus, and only in a certain subset of tinnitus sufferers. One study found that the drug gabapentin was successful in reducing tinnitus annoyance amongst patients who had tinnitus due to an exposure to loud noise, but the drug had no effect on the control group consisting of patients with tinnitus that was not a result of exposure to loud noise[69]. Such results make any recommendation for gabapentin use highly specific to a particular group of tinnitus sufferers. However, another study found that a slightly lower dose of gabapentin over time had no effect on tinnitus[70].

For the most part, other medications including antihistamines, vasodilators, barbiturates, and muscle relaxers, have all been studied for their potential benefits in the improvement of tinnitus. Unfortunately, none showed much of any promise under the conditions studied[71]. As a result of the relative lack of benefit from medications for the treatment of tinnitus, guidelines put out by the American Academy of Otolaryngology – Head and Neck Surgery Foundation (AAO-HNS) lists medication use for the treatment of tinnitus as a treatment that they do not recommend[12].

Despite the lack of endorsement of medication by the AAO-HNS, one point should be noted when it comes to pharmaceuticals and tinnitus. While the general conclusion is that drug treatment has relatively little if any effect on improving tinnitus, it has been discussed that the fact that some drugs can *cause* tinnitus suggests a potential target for future research[60]. If the structure and action of drugs that cause tinnitus can be studied in depth, it may reveal new insights into the mechanism involved in the generation of tinnitus. Therefore, drug therapy should not necessarily be counted out but instead must be considered as a further opportunity for the study of tinnitus.

Dietary supplement treatment for tinnitus

Though not as prevalent as drug research, there has been some scientific investigation into supplement use for the treatment of tinnitus. Much like pharmaceutical treatments, the results are not particularly promising, yet the wealth of available supplements along with the promise of those yet to be discovered do suggest that supplements may be a source of help for tinnitus sufferers.

Vitamin B12 has been targeted as a potential vitamin-based treatment due to the fact that deficiencies can have a negative effect on nerve tissue. One study determined that a few subjects found a bit of relief from tinnitus after intramuscular injection of B12, but the results were not consistent across participants[72].

The use of zinc has been suggested to help tinnitus as a result of its role in maintenance of the nervous system[12]. However, one study investigating its effects in elderly patients found no real change in loudness or annoyance of tinnitus. Furthermore, indigestion was reported as a side effect from the zinc treatment[73].

Ginkgo biloba has been targeted as a potential treatment for tinnitus and over the years has become the most popular supplement for the treatment of tinnitus[12]. While there have been somewhat mixed results specific to ginkgo biloba's effects on tinnitus[74], most studies looking at the reported effects have been said to suffer from flaws in the study design[12]. Therefore, much like pharmaceutical use in the treatment of tinnitus, the AAO-HNS does not endorse the use of gingko biloba or any other supplement[12].

Sound therapy

First conducted in the 1970s, treating tinnitus through the use of sound therapy involves the production of an audible tone that effectively cancels out, or 'masks' the tinnitus[75]. The purpose of masking is to both manage a patient's reaction to tinnitus as well as reduce the perception of tinnitus[12].

It is thought that sound therapy influences tinnitus in several ways. First, it serves to reduce the vast perceived difference between a patient's tinnitus and the environment[76]. Sound therapy can also provide soothing sounds that reduce a patient's stress brought on by tinnitus[77], or provide sound in such a way that it distracts the patient from their ongoing tinnitus[77]. You may have used sound therapy if you have tried one of those white noise generators that play sounds such as waves, wind, or soft music. Sound generators come in many forms and may be quite large such as an alarm clock or wearable in the form of a hearing aid, including some hearing aids that include built-in sound generators[11].

A more specific type of sound therapy involves personalized sound stimulation. This type of treatment uses sound to attempt to 'fill in the gaps' of where a person's hearing loss occurs[78]. There is also a similar type of sound therapy that generates music in the frequency of the tinnitus[79].

While sound generators may have the ability to distract or cover up a patient's tinnitus during use, there remains a lack of evidence supporting sound therapy as a viable treatment for tinnitus[12]. More specifically, it has been noted that sound therapy *alone* does not have much effect; however, it has been suggested that sound therapy may have an improved benefit when used in conjunction with other tinnitus therapies[80].

Counseling

Though not necessarily a 'treatment' in the sense that it does not attempt to improve a patient's tinnitus directly, counseling can help the patient adjust to their tinnitus diagnosis, in turn helping alleviate some of the associated conditions such as stress or anxiety. The counseling typically involves providing information and advice to the patient that can help the patient accept and become accustomed to their existing tinnitus[11]. Components of counseling include coping mechanisms to deal with tinnitus-related issues such as emotional distress, difficulties in sleeping, concentration and attention difficulties, and impact on their personal and social lives[11]. Unlike other behavioral therapies, counseling focuses more on helping the patient get through the stresses associated with their tinnitus. While there are few quality studies that investigate the effects of counseling alone as a therapy for tinnitus, it is generally accepted that psychological counseling is an essential and beneficial aspect of managing tinnitus[11, 15].

Cognitive Behavioral Therapy

The use of cognitive behavioral therapy (CBT) is to refocus generally negative thoughts about tinnitus into a more positive view[12]. Typically, CBT training requires sessions with a mental health professional for one to two hours per session and lasting anywhere from 8-24 weeks[12]. More recently, CBT training has become available via the internet, providing a less-costly option for patients as well as a less time-intensive session for therapists[12]. Furthermore, internet-based CBT appears to have similar positive effects as traditional face-to-face counseling[81]. Tinnitus is well-known to trigger depressive thoughts, and the basis of CBT is to help identify the main negative factors in those thoughts and try to make them more positive.

For example, if a tinnitus patient feels that an invitation to a concert would be a waste of time due to not hearing the distinct sounds of the music, CBT would attempt to restructure that generally negative thought into one that helps the patient focus more on enjoying time with friends, finding the most acoustic-friendly seats, and maybe adding additional activities that would be more conducive to making the time enjoyable. Or, perhaps the therapy would trigger the idea to have the patient drive herself to the concert so as to avoid the unfortunate situation of feeling like she needs to stay due to needing a ride home. Additional CBT treatments might include relaxation therapies to use on the way to the concert, taking a nap prior to the concert to cut down on the occurrence of fatigue, and ways to perhaps improve her experience at the concert such as wearing an earplug to reduce excessively loud noise.

Alternatively, a patient newly-diagnosed with tinnitus may have difficulty getting out of bed each morning due to depression related to his tinnitus. A CBT-based therapy may include setting goals the prior evening regarding what can be accomplished the next day in order to both motivate the patient to get started and also – if the goals are met – give the patient a feeling of accomplishment at the end of the day.

The evidence is quite favorable for CBT in relation to tinnitus, and as such the AAO-HNS recommends CBT for the treatment of tinnitus. Most often, the benefit of CBT is not in the reduction of the tinnitus noise but rather in an improvement in the patient's quality of life[82, 83]. It has been reported that CBT was shown to be more effective than counseling alone[84]. Yet, one study reported that when CBT was combined with counseling there was a decrease in tinnitus severity and impairment as well as an improvement in quality of life[85].

Invasive therapies

In outlining the various invasive treatment options, we will limit our discussion of invasive tinnitus therapy to acupuncture and surgery. Intravenous or intratympanic injections have been discussed in the pharmaceutical section and will not be outlined here.

Acupuncture is a widely-used therapy that involves the placement of thin needles in specific areas of the body. Specific to tinnitus, the research highlights conflicting levels of success in response to acupuncture. One study reported that acupuncture had a greater effect on tinnitus than prescription medication[86]. However, this study and many more were reported to have issues with their experimental design, in turn calling into question the validity of any positive (or negative) result of acupuncture for the treatment of tinnitus[87]. As a result, the AAO-HNS does not recommend acupuncture as a viable option for the treatment of tinnitus[12].

Surgery as a treatment option for the sole symptom of tinnitus does not exist. However, several ear conditions exist for which surgery is an option, and those conditions may have tinnitus as an associated symptom[88]. When surgery is an option for these other medical conditions, tinnitus can be assessed post-surgery to determine if there was an improvement. For example, tympanoplasty – reconstruction of the eardrum – has been reported to improve tinnitus and satisfaction in two-thirds of patients[89]. Conversely, shunt insertion and/or cutting of the vestibular nerve – both treatment options for Ménière's disease – have been reported to have no effect on tinnitus[90]. Based on the available research, a patient should not expect an improvement in his or her tinnitus as a result of surgery for another inner-ear condition.

Alternative treatments

Conduct a quick internet search for options available to treat tinnitus and you will get highly variable and wide-ranging responses. Just typing in the words "tinnitus treatment" (with quotes) into a search engine returns both medical-based websites as well as at-home treatments. These medical pages can be informative, but it is important as a consumer and patient to evaluate the source of that information. Think back to what we discussed earlier in this chapter about a case versus a pool of subjects. If a webpage you are reading touts a particular product for tinnitus but is actually an individual's personal blog, there is a reduced chance that you will find references outlining either the source of their information or any evidence of how their product has been properly tested on tinnitus patients.

Many, many other alternative treatments exist out there. Magnets, essential oils, and green tea extract are all hailed by some as tinnitus treatments – often on social media or discussion boards that rely only on anecdotal evidence rather than any scientific basis. If you want more information about those products, certainly send the individual a message or post a reply seeking references and/or resources. Search for product reviews and read what others have to say about the item. Or, conduct your own internet search for the specific product or idea. The premise in doing so is to maximize your efforts in finding ways to reduce your tinnitus and improve your quality of life. Given that some treatments are described as taking months or more to see an effect, it is important that you separate the viable alternative treatments from the shams.

For example, searching for *homeopathic remedies for tinnitus* returned the following products (among many others):

Calcarea carbonica	Kali carbonicum
Calcarea fluor	Lycopodium
China	Natrum salicylicum
Chinium sulph	Psorinum
Cimicifuga	Salicylicum acidum
Coffee cruda	Silicea
Conium maculatum	Tellurium metallicum
Graphites	

If you have time, conduct a search for each product and look for scientific studies that test the effects of each item on tinnitus. I am guessing you will not find much in the way of strong evidence. As a consumer, you must ask yourself why that is, or why the medical community is not touting the benefits of each and every tinnitus product you see advertised. You'll likely find that there's a lack of supporting evidence, and most medical professionals won't recommend a product to you without seeing viable evidence, which most of these products cannot claim. That is not to say that the products don't work; rather, there's not a lot of evidence that consistently points towards positive effects with tinnitus. You may have success, and if other proven treatments aren't working – and there are no harmful side effects – it probably won't hurt to try.

I am not by any means disputing any of these homeopathic or alternative treatment products for the treatment of tinnitus. Remember back to the earlier portion of this chapter that until a cure exists for tinnitus, *all* available options and treatments must be evaluated. However, I want to ensure that you as a consumer and a patient are not taken advantage of, either. Ask yourself what evidence supports the use of these alternative remedies. Determine whether each product is supposed to cure or treat tinnitus, and if it is to treat tinnitus, to what degree should someone expect improvement? These and many other questions are important to consider, as you don't want to be taken advantage of as a consumer. Furthermore, if you have new or severe tinnitus your newfound frustration with tinnitus may make you somewhat eager to purchase a product that you are told will stop your tinnitus, when in fact you should be quite hesitant and inquisitive instead.

Be sure to take time to evaluate the evidence as well as the claims associated with any product (pharmaceutical, homeopathic, etc.) you are considering. For example, one homeopathic website noted that a patient reported a 10% decrease in tinnitus after one month, and a big decrease in the perception of tinnitus after six months of using a product. As a researcher myself, I would have several questions specific to this type of testimonial. First, how can one measure a 10% difference in tinnitus other than by what the patient states. For example, if you are inside a quiet room – where your tinnitus is likely more noticeable – and then step outside to a non-enclosed area where your senses are somewhat distracted, couldn't you expect a 10% decrease immediately in your tinnitus, even without consuming the product? And, as a consumer, is the price of the product worth a 10% decrease in your tinnitus? I would also want to see more data that one customer reporting a 10% decrease in his or her tinnitus.

Second, the website touts that the patient reports a 10% decrease in tinnitus followed by a 'big decrease' in *perception* of tinnitus. In my opinion, those are two different aspects. So, the seller would have to convince me that their product influences the perception of tinnitus as much as it influences tinnitus. Several therapies can help reduce tinnitus perception by distracting from the tinnitus, and over time it is expected that a patient becomes 'used to' his or her tinnitus. Therefore, any decrease in perception of tinnitus after six months could be a normal expectation of the timeline of having tinnitus rather than being due to any homeopathic treatment (think back to the coincidence we discussed earlier in this chapter).

The 'tapping' treatment

I wouldn't be honest as an author if I didn't include one more treatment for tinnitus that I stumbled across. There's one thing, though, that separates this treatment from all others – it worked. I have seen it called by various names including the 'finger tapping' or 'finger drumming' technique, and it involves a series of tapping movements against the back of the skull. What is important to note though is that although I say that it worked for my tinnitus – along with several other testimonials found online – the results were only temporary.

To perform the maneuver, place your elbows on a desk and then place the palm of your hands over your ears. Spread your fingers out around the back of your head so that the tips of your fingers are approximately one inch apart, and then place your index finger on top of your middle finger. You're your index finger, apply pressure against the middle finger so that your index finger slides off and 'snaps' forcefully against the back of your head. You should feel a significant tap on your skull. Repeat this every second or so, approximately 50 times.

When I did this maneuver, my tinnitus was gone. Not reduced, but *gone.* It lasted about ten minutes or so, and then slowly returned to its normal level. Online there are similar reports of people who claim instant relief as well, though not everyone claims to have success with this technique.

Part of the problem in recommending such a procedure is that there is no rational explanation that outlines why the technique works. This is immediately countered by someone like me with the statement *but it WORKS*. Such a rationale goes back to what we discussed before in that even though there's not necessarily a viable explanation, if there is no harm done then it may be a worthwhile treatment.

In conclusion

Without a cure for the annoyance of tinnitus, we are left only with treatments to help us deal with tinnitus. As treatments are studied for their viability in improving tinnitus, those treatments that don't show a consistent effect are largely eliminated from the discussion over time. While the elimination of any treatment may seem somewhat detrimental, it can in fact be a positive event as it leaves only those treatments that show promise. Consumers – in this case tinnitus patients – can then weigh the benefits of a treatment against any potential cost, whether that cost be financial or emotional.

It must be remembered that for the most part, tinnitus treatments are focused on psychological tactics that work to improve a patient's quality of life. Pharmaceutical treatments have shown some promise, but one major roadblock to finding an effective pharmacological treatment is that we don't yet know the intricate structures that cause our tinnitus. Medicines typically rely on an interaction between the drug molecule and small tissue-specific proteins, and given that we have not yet identified which tissues are directly responsible for tinnitus, we cannot adequately develop tinnitus medicines given that we do not yet know which tissue(s) to target.

In lieu of the structured, scientifically-tested tinnitus treatments, we still have our homeopathic and alternative treatment options for battling our tinnitus. When it comes to these 'non-traditional' or 'non-scientific' treatments, the patient and/or caregiver should ask themselves one question: *if a patient reports relief from tinnitus treatment that does not have a favorable endorsement from the scientific community, should that treatment be continued*? If there is no real risk to the patient and the treatment is affordable, it is difficult to say that the treatment should not be continued. The tinnitus patient must remain aware, though, that there are many 'gimmick' treatments out there, and the anecdotal nature by which some treatments are reported as "successful" can be frustrating.

In the case of tinnitus, which is merely a symptom of some other, possibly harmless condition, reporting the success of *all* treatments is warranted if no harm is to be expected as a result of the application of the treatment. Some might argue that from an ethical standpoint, a medical practitioner or caregiver may be entering onto shaky ground should he or she suggest that a patient stop a treatment that shows benefit for the patient despite any viable scientific backing.

The anecdotal nature of so many tinnitus treatments is precisely why I included the section on the scientific process at the beginning of this chapter. It was certainly not to bore you with details. Rather, it was to help you think like a scientist in order to evaluate the quality of the available evidence and to make informed decisions as both a patient and a consumer. This approach should apply to all treatment options – not just homeopathic. Take special caution when presented with homeopathic treatments that cost money, as a thorough evaluation of the evidence – from the seller to the ingredients to the treatment's theory – should be conducted. When armed with the right information for all tinnitus treatments, you can become not only a more informed patient but also ensure that your efforts are focused on the most appropriate treatment for your tinnitus.

Chapter 6: Associated conditions

A S WE HAVE DISCUSSED, tinnitus is a symptom associated with a separate medical condition rather than being a true medical condition itself. Therefore, in the case of chronic tinnitus there is usually a primary medical condition that triggers tinnitus as a symptom. This underlying condition may be as simple as age-associated degeneration of hearing structures or repeated exposure to loud noise, or it can be more complicated such as might occur with an inner ear tumor or Ménière's disease. While there are many conditions (e.g. high blood pressure) that can occur throughout the body that have been associated with tinnitus, in this chapter we will largely focus on those conditions specific to the immediate area around the ear. In reading about these medical conditions and their ability to trigger tinnitus, you will hopefully recognize the importance of getting a thorough medical evaluation upon noticing persistent tinnitus, particularly if the tinnitus has been present for a while and/or is not associated with an exposure to an unusually loud noise like gunfire or a concert.

Minor conditions

Several relatively minor conditions of the ear can influence tinnitus. In temporary conditions such as ear wax buildup or a tear of the eardrum, the associated tinnitus will probably diminish or be eliminated upon addressing the affected issue (e.g. healing of the eardrum). Even though many causes of tinnitus can be extremely minor, it is essential that all cases of tinnitus be evaluated by a medical professional. In the event that the tinnitus cause is minor, the medical professional will likely be able to address the issue such as through removal of impacted ear wax or diagnosing a tear in the eardrum and prescribing proper treatment which should in turn reduce the impact of the tinnitus.

Medication use

If you read the side effects of almost any drug, there's a good chance that you'll see "ringing of the ears" somewhere on the list. While many of the reports of tinnitus associated with prescription or over-the-counter drugs are valid, it should be understood that some reported side effects are listed in part because tinnitus was reported during the drug testing phase. It may be that the subject had faint ringing in his or her ears before the drug test but didn't recognize it, and when asked "do you notice ringing in your ears" after taking the drug, it was suddenly realized that there was a bit of tinnitus. Despite a general lack of true association, tinnitus would nonetheless go down as a noted side effect, even if it wasn't *specifically* tied to the use of that particular drug. Therefore, even though some drugs are associated with tinnitus, don't automatically assume that if you take the drug you will get or have worsening of your tinnitus.

There are a few drugs that have a higher rate of triggering or aggravating tinnitus and possibly hearing loss. These drug classes (not drug *names*) include the following: certain non-steroidal anti-inflammatory drugs (NSAIDs), some antibiotics (e.g. aminoglycosides), quinine, certain diuretics, and at least one cancer drug (cisplatin)[23].

Many drugs, such as certain NSAIDs, can induce tinnitus during the time frame that the drug is being taken. As such, when the drug therapy is stopped, the tinnitus generally disappears soon after stopping the drug[60]. It should be noted though that certain drugs are ototoxic and can harm the ear tissue when taken at certain doses. Therefore, it is important when taking medication to discuss your tinnitus with your doctor and notify him or her of any possible changes.

Otosclerosis

Otosclerosis is an abnormal growth of tissue within the inner ear that affects from 0.2-2.1% of the adult population[91] and is approximately twice as common in women as men[23]. Typically, patients affected by otosclerosis are affected in both ears[92], and tinnitus is a common symptom.

It is thought that otosclerosis influences tinnitus through either hearing loss that results in reduced environmental sounds (and thereby amplifies tinnitus), abnormal blood flow[93], or potentially through enzymatic damage induced by degeneration of the cochlear bone[23].

Several treatments are available for otosclerosis, including hearing aid use, treatment with sodium fluoride, and surgical intervention[23]. After surgery, 64% of patients have reported elimination of tinnitus in comparison to no change (14%) or worsening tinnitus (6%)[94], all with no apparent effect on hearing. Another study found similar results after stapes bone surgery resulting from otosclerosis. There, of 74% of patients reporting tinnitus prior to surgery, 60% of those patients claimed that their tinnitus was eliminated after surgery, with just 8.8% and 2.9% reporting unchanged or worsened tinnitus post-surgery[95].

Ménière's disease

Ménière's disease is a condition thought to result from problems with the fluid regulation system of the inner ear. Ménière's patients typically experience an ongoing degree of unsteadiness and ear pressure or fullness intermixed with bouts of acute vertigo, nausea, and vomiting that can last several hours or more. Tinnitus is also a common problem for Ménière's patients[96]. Due in large part to the complexity and sensitivity of the vestibular system, Ménière's remains a complicated disease. While the acute vertigo attacks of Ménière's can be extremely debilitating, these attacks can be followed by months or years of almost no symptoms.

Several theorized causes of Ménière's have been proposed, including body water regulation issues, endolymph reabsorption anomalies, vascular abnormalities, and autoimmune factors. Of these possible causes, fluid regulation in the middle ear is considered to be one of the main triggers of Ménière's[97]. For example, water channels, which regulate the transport of water across membranes, have been implicated as a possible main cause of Meniere's[98]. This theory results from the idea that unexpected reductions or increases in the number of water channels can influence the balance of fluid on each side of a membrane, and any alteration fluid balance can have negative consequences in the equilibrium system of the ear.

Similarly, some researchers suggest that Ménière's patients have a diminished capacity to regulate fluid within their inner ear[99]. Consequently, fluctuations in the inner ear fluid are not well tolerated in Ménière's patients. This is thought to lead to fluid imbalances that contribute to many of the symptoms encountered by Ménière's patients. Electrolytes such as sodium that are known to play a role in the body's fluid regulation are commonly restricted in Ménière's patients in order to reduce potential fluctuations within the middle ear.

Other theorized causes of Ménière's disease include autoimmune disorders[100], the herpes virus[101], cervical (i.e. neck) disorders[102] and stress[103]. Whereas no definitive cause of Ménière's has been discovered, it is vital that research continue to investigate these and all logical possibilities to determine the potential link between Ménière's and tinnitus. At present there remains no cure for Ménière's, though symptoms can often be controlled through the aforementioned sodium restriction as well as through medication, intratympanic steroid injection, and if necessary, surgical procedures on the middle ear.

Temporomandibular joint disorder

Temporomandibular joint (TMJ) disorder is a relatively common condition affecting up to 20% of the adult population[23]. Individuals with TMJ typically report pain in the area of the TMJ, located just in front of the outer ear canal. Although the TMJ and ear are located immediately next to each other, it has been reported that any simultaneous occurrence of tinnitus and TMJ disorder are pure chance[104]. Still, others have suggested that the high rate of TMJ in conjunction with tinnitus indicates that there is a potential link between the two conditions[105]. For example, one study looked at 20 patients with tinnitus but no reports of TMJ or evident ear issues. However, when x-rays were taken and further tests conducted, 19 of those 20 patients were found to have some form of detectable TMJ disorder[106]. This suggests that at least in some patients there is an underlying, previously undetected TMJ condition in patients exhibiting tinnitus. Yet, others have suggested that TMJ-associated tinnitus may be due to large doses of anti-inflammatory drugs being used to treat the TMJ[107].

Treatment for TMJ is relatively straightforward and includes anti-inflammatory drugs, adherence to a soft diet to avoid excessive or forceful chewing, and possible use of oral splints.

Surgery is typically only recommended in the event that one of these treatments has failed[23].

Acoustic Neuroma

Acoustic neuromas are slow growing benign tumors[108] that grow on the nerve tissue of the eighth (vestibulocochlear) nerve[109]. Reports indicate that anywhere from 75-100% of individuals with neuromas have tinnitus, and the neuroma itself is typically discovered when the patient is initially evaluated for tinnitus[16, 110]. Several theories as to how acoustic neuromas trigger tinnitus have been proposed. One suggests that as the tumor grows larger it takes up space within the nerve, thereby compressing the nerve fibers and causing the individual fibers to inadvertently 'talk' to each other[111]. Another theory suggests a multitude of possibly cochlear issues[112], while a third explanation suggests that tinnitus arises from within the brain[113]. The belief is still held that there are most likely multiple issues involved in the link between acoustic neuromas and tinnitus[112].

Treatment for an acoustic neuroma can range from conservative methods such as observation to the more intensive use of radiation[114] and/or surgical removal[109, 115].

Other associated conditions

A quick internet search will reveal a variety of other, non-ear-related medical conditions suspected to cause chronic tinnitus. Examples include diabetes, dementia, kidney disease, or even heart attacks. While not to downplay the validity of these reports, I recommend that you are diligent in evaluating the source of these claims and understand that because you have tinnitus it is not any sort of guarantee that you have one of these medical conditions. Only a thorough medical evaluation – preferably with a specialist trained in the various conditions of the ear – will tell you whether a source for your tinnitus can be determined.

I should also point out that many web results discussing tinnitus-related conditions often include a product for sale which is almost always described as beneficial or even essential for eliminating your tinnitus. Be aware of this tactic, and refer back to the scientific process that we discussed in the tinnitus treatment chapter to help you discern the difference between reliable information and outright scams. As we have discussed previously, tinnitus can be a very frustrating condition, and patients are often willing to do seemingly anything to stop the annoying phantom sound in their ears. Always take the time to get a thorough medical evaluation to look for all possible causes of the tinnitus, and talk with your medical provider about the best treatment options for your particular situation.

Chapter 7: Tinnitus and Quality of Life

DESPITE ITS PREVALENCE and at times overpowering effects, tinnitus remains just a symptom and therefore has no real effect on an individual's physical health. However, tinnitus has been shown to have a significant impact on a patient's quality of life. Tinnitus can prompt events such as anxiety, stress, or anger, which often result in physical manifestations such as elevated blood pressure, increased stress hormones, or other events. Therefore, understanding the effect that tinnitus has on an individual's quality of life may help alleviate some of these concerns.

Tinnitus is a symptom much like pain. Both are harmless in and of themselves but can have extreme influence on our daily life. Think about it – when you have pain, you address it. It may be relatively minor and you just 'push through it', but even if it's minor but turns chronic in nature, most likely you will eventually receive medical attention to address the cause of the pain. You may have even heard that old saying of "pain is good", referring to the body's use of pain to alert us to an underlying problem.

With tinnitus, however, even though you want to address it as you would with pain, no current treatment is known that will terminate the tinnitus. Addressing the cause of the pain might involve medication (e.g. anti-inflammatories), rehabilitation, or surgery, and typically there is a significant reduction if not elimination of the pain. With tinnitus, however, even though it is associated with an underlying medical condition we have no current way to eliminate or even significantly reduce its effects. This naturally causes a source of anxiety for patients with tinnitus, and is heightened by the fact that we cannot do anything to eliminate the tinnitus. Therefore, an initial diagnosis of chronic tinnitus can lead to misrepresented fears such as the tinnitus worsening, a further diminished loss of hearing, and potentially thoughts of becoming completely deaf. These type of thoughts are typically what leads to a reduced quality of life for tinnitus sufferers.

Because tinnitus is a symptom, it is not physical in the sense of an ankle sprain or a nerve impingement. There is as of yet no 'quick fix' to help us alleviate the ringing sound in our ears. As we have discussed, a large portion of people who have noticeable tinnitus do not seek medical treatment for the condition[15]. Because tinnitus does not have any outward physical signs, medical practitioners must rely upon what is reported by the patient, and descriptions of just what is occurring can unfortunately vary greatly between patients. Furthermore, patients with certain conditions such as high blood pressure or diabetes report a lower quality of life score than otherwise healthy patients[116].

Tinnitus' impact on quality of life can also vary greatly between patients. One might argue that any presence of long-term tinnitus is detrimental, as being in any quiet environment is likely to be interrupted by the constant sound of tinnitus. This might occur when trying to relax in a quiet room, or when taking a test, or when going to sleep, each of which is a condition that typically calls for minimal sound intrusion. The addition of tinnitus to the environment could result in a failure to relax, or perhaps a reduction in sleep quality brought about by a difficulty in falling asleep. This may in turn result in fatigue the following day which can affect awareness as well as mood, thereby indirectly affecting those who interact with the patient[117].

These indirect complications of tinnitus can have a significant impact on a tinnitus sufferer's life. So much so that in 2007 the World Health Organization (WHO) researched how tinnitus influences quality of life and used the resulting findings to establish four areas that were negatively affected by tinnitus: thoughts and emotions, hearing, sleep, and concentration[118]. The WHO reported that when these areas were affected there were additional indirect factors that were also influenced that could in turn further impact a patient's quality of life. Therefore, even though medical treatment may not be sought for tinnitus, there is likely some degree of intrusion upon each patient's life and potentially the lives of others.

It has been reported that personality characteristics can predispose a tinnitus patient to have what they describe as 'distressing' tinnitus[15]. Similarly, a patient's response to their tinnitus has been shown to affect their interaction with others and can heighten their stress level in a way that in turn affects activities such as driving, eating, or performing tasks[119]. Much of the detrimental effects on quality of life associated with tinnitus have been reported to stem from both the difficulty in curing tinnitus and in an inability to outline an underlying tinnitus cause[120].

Along these same lines, there is a common rate of psychiatric conditions reported in patients with tinnitus[12]. For example, depression is reported in up to 60% of tinnitus patients[121], and a patient's level of depression has been shown to be related to the degree of tinnitus[122]. However, the balance between depression and tinnitus is not well understood.

Researchers are not clear as to whether tinnitus causes depression, whether depression influences the tinnitus, or if depression leads to the development of tinnitus[123].

Interestingly, it was found that patients who exhibited a "Type D" personality were more apt to be negatively affected by tinnitus, including higher rates of anxiety and depression as well as reporting tinnitus-related distress[124]. Type D personalities are considered a 'distressed' personality type[125] and reflect a unique combination of tending to experience negative emotions in conjunction with a likelihood of not expressing emotions due to fear of rejection by others. If both of these traits exist, the individual is classified as a Type D personality[125]. This is important, as tinnitus itself is adept at causing depression, and in an individual likely to suppress emotions *and* experience negative emotions often, it can be a volatile mix. Therefore, medical intervention may be necessary for these type of individuals.

As far back as 1983, when the first effects of tinnitus on quality of life were reported, patients noted insomnia, difficulty in understanding speech, depression, difficulty concentrating, and issues involving both family and work life[126]. Since then, additional research has found that tinnitus-related issues have not changed much. However, one recent study reported that when compared to non-tinnitus sufferers who had only hearing loss, tinnitus patients

109

reported higher levels of stress, lower social closeness, lower self-control, and higher alienation[127]. This research indicates that tinnitus further escalates any impairment to quality of life as compared to other benign ear-related issues such as hearing deficits.

More recent research was conducted on a very broad group of patients with a high degree of diversity in their degree of tinnitus[128]. The study looked at self-reported tinnitus and its effect on quality of life and depression. The results found that the biggest influence between quality of life and depression were from the following conditions: feeling confused from tinnitus, the trouble of falling asleep at night, the interference with job or household responsibilities, getting upset from tinnitus, and the feeling of being depressed. Interestingly, factors including concentration difficulties, hearing difficulties, interference with social relationships and activities, irritability, frustration, lack of control and escape, and angriness were all found to be unrelated to their quality of life and depression scores. This research contradicts many other study findings, yet reflects well the variability often associated with tinnitus research.

Physical activity engagement has been shown to correlate with improved health-related quality of life[129]. Gender has been shown to play a role in some studies, yet the results are quite inconsistent. One study found that women reported being more annoyed by tinnitus than males[130] while others have shown that males report more annoyance[131, 132]. Still, other findings report no difference in the influence of tinnitus between males and females[33].

Quality of life appears to be influenced by the length of time that the patient has had tinnitus. One study found that tinnitus had a stronger impact in patients who had experienced tinnitus less than five years than in patients who had tinnitus more than five years[133]. This suggests that there is an initial problem in coping with tinnitus that seems to fade over time such that quality of life becomes less impacted. This fits well with what we have discussed previously – that most people experiencing chronic tinnitus eventually adapt to the tinnitus in their ear and lead relatively normal lives[120]. Furthermore, research has shown that patients who have higher tinnitus 'acceptance' scores report a higher quality of life as well as lower psychological distress[134].

Even though older adults are more commonly affected by tinnitus, they are not immune to the decreased quality of life that can result. One study surveying older adults reported that having severe tinnitus resulted in a "Role-Physical" quality of life (i.e. the degree to which one's health results in a diminished ability to perform activities at work or home) similar to that of a non-tinnitus patient experiencing congestive heart failure[135]. Furthermore, the Bodily Pain index, which assesses the quantity and effect of pain in the body over the prior four weeks) was reported to score worse for older adults with tinnitus than non-tinnitus patients with either chronic, obstructive pulmonary disease (COPD) or high blood pressure. And, as has been shown to occur in a younger population[122], this older population reported that their use of antidepressant medication increased as the degree of tinnitus increased.

In conclusion

Clearly, tinnitus can have a significant impact on a sufferer's quality of life. Yet, because tinnitus is a symptom, there is no specific physical harm occurring to the body that is directly related to tinnitus. However, as there can be a distressing psychological impact from tinnitus, it is important that patients take action to address the many psychological issues that can arise as a result of tinnitus such as depression or anxiety. Research has consistently shown that quality of life scores can improve when a patient is proactive about addressing his or her tinnitus. This can in turn result in an improvement in overall health as well.

Chapter 8: Life with a tinnitus sufferer

IF YOU HAVE NEVER EXPERIENCED tinnitus, even the temporary kind that exists for a few days after a loud event such as a concert, it can be somewhat difficult to understand the annoyance and frustration that tinnitus can bring. If, on the other hand you have had even a temporary bout of tinnitus, you might remember that high-pitched or howling sound in your ear that lasted a day or two. Imagine now that the sound exists *constantly* and *does not stop* at all. That is life with chronic tinnitus.

When I wrote this book, it was designed to be a resource for both those people living with tinnitus and those that care for people with tinnitus whether it be a spouse, parent, or friend. This chapter focuses on that latter group – those that don't have tinnitus but live or interact with someone that does. Because it can be difficult to grasp the frustrations and challenges involved with tinnitus, I wrote this chapter to outline some potential tips for making tinnitus tolerable for both you and the patient. Keep in mind that the focus of this chapter is not based on scientific studies but rather a culmination of stories I have read along with my own personal experience. Your interaction with a tinnitus sufferer may be very similar yet could also be vastly different.

Hearing

As you've read in this book, tinnitus is very often associated with age-related hearing loss. This has a two-fold effect on the patient's ability to hear. Not only is his or her hearing diminished, but there is also a new 'noise' in their ear as well. So the patient has a dual negative effect – it is harder for them to hear, and what they do hear has to occur over an ever-present perceived sound – both of which combine to make hearing things like normal conversation much more difficult. Throw in a bit of background sound and listening to conversation becomes even more difficult. You will probably notice that the patient asks you to repeat things more often. In particular, if there is ample environmental noise such as outdoor sounds (i.e. traffic, wind, etc.) or background conversation such as might occur in a crowded room, it is likely going to be very difficult for the tinnitus sufferer to hear *and comprehend* what you are saying. Expect to have to speak louder and more distinctly in order that they can receive and process your conversation.

One thing that I can tell you after having both experienced tinnitus and having read a lot of material in preparation for this book is that the tinnitus patient hates to be reminded of his or her condition. Therefore, both because tinnitus can fluctuate and because background noise can vary, it is best to not assume that the patient cannot hear you. Talking loud and distinctly at a small gathering may be unnecessary, in turn drawing the attention of everyone around and likely putting the tinnitus patient 'on the spot'. Therefore, work to converse with any tinnitus sufferer normally, but expect to have to repeat yourself a few times as the environment changes.

Frustration

Whether the tinnitus exists due to an accident, chronic exposure to loud sounds, or just age-related hearing loss, expect that with the initial phases of tinnitus there will be a lot of frustration and aggravation from the patient. This new, constant sound in his or her ear can be deafening at times, and even when it's not deafening, it's still there. It's there when they sleep, when they wake up, and it's interrupting every fun or bothersome event that they participate in. For many, sleep may be their only reprieve from the tinnitus.

Consequently, because of the constant presence of the tinnitus there is no escape. When they are sick of it, it's still there. Therefore, because they are already agitated from their tinnitus, expect that any little interruption or setback will annoy, anger, or frustrate them further, perhaps even more than it would have prior to their tinnitus. Over time, as the patient applies various treatments and hopefully grows accustomed to the ever-present tinnitus, you will hopefully see a reduction in this frustration as the tinnitus becomes less and less bothersome. The hardest time for you as a caregiver will likely be those initial months of tinnitus, when it can seem unbearable for the patient. If you can make it through the initial phases, you will hopefully see a significant change in the patient's ability to deal with the tinnitus.

A large degree of how much frustration you'll notice may well be related to the patient's personality. A very outgoing, vocal individual will in most cases be more apt to discuss and point out their frustration. Conversely, a quieter, perhaps more introverted individual may largely keep his or her tinnitus-related frustration to themselves. When this quieter type of individual has an outburst of frustration – such as when they can't hear the television or a phone conversation – it is typically a bit more unexpected than a similar outburst from someone who is more vocal about their tinnitus. You as the caregiver must try to remember this and put their outburst into context – they are not angry at you; rather, they are almost certain to be frustrated with not hearing the same conversation they likely could hear prior to their tinnitus.

Noisy environments

Along the lines of having issues with hearing, noisy environments can be problematic for the tinnitus sufferer. Dinner dates, social events, and outdoor conversations are all situations that can make hearing and comprehension difficult for a tinnitus sufferer. The amount of effort it can take to piece together a simple conversation in each of these situations can be quite fatiguing, and in many cases can be impossible. In my case, when in a loud environment during my initial time with tinnitus I would often piece together a conversation using keywords that I could pick up from the other person. I tried as hard as I could to avoid asking the dreaded *"what?"* question, when in reality I would often wish that I could ask that after almost every sentence.

If you are with a tinnitus sufferer, when presented with an opportunity to attend an event in a noisy environment you should assume a bit of hesitation on his or her part. Expect that their mind is calculating out the positive and negative aspects of accepting the offer, which may be ranging from "a chance to spend some quiet time with my wife" to "everyone's going to be annoyed that I'm there". Avoid viewing this mindset as selfishness on their part; instead, try to understand that what you might see as a nice dinner with friends could easily be viewed by a tinnitus sufferer as another reminder that they cannot hear, they are a burden to those around them, and/or they have lost their ability to enjoy the company of others. It might seem extreme, but when you live with tinnitus you have a different view of social events.

Quiet environments

Strangely enough, tinnitus has a way of affecting the extremes of a person's interaction with their environment. Noisy situations result in an inability of the tinnitus sufferer to hear the intricacies of a conversation while quiet situations make the tinnitus itself seem overpowering.

Understand that the definition of 'quiet' is somewhat subjective. Some may view sitting on the couch and reading a good book as 'peace and quiet'. To a tinnitus sufferer though, that scenario may be unbearable as it is 'too' quiet. Instead, he or she may turn the television (or some other device) on as it can provide an ambient amount of noise that allows them to comfortably do something like read a book. What many sufferers dread is the *dead silent* situation, such as typically occurs when lying in bed trying to go to sleep. When there is an absence of background noise, the perceived sound of tinnitus can be overwhelming, starting a vicious cycle of adding stress, which may increase the sound of the tinnitus, which increases the patient's stress, and so on.

Therefore, many tinnitus sufferers will utilize a background noise to help drown out the tinnitus. Some prefer to have a television on, while others like white noise such as that of a fan. Even though I can effectively drown out my tinnitus I still prefer to sleep with the background sound of a ceiling fan, but that is based upon my own type and degree of tinnitus. Others with a different type or severity of tinnitus may say that the fan is not loud enough and require an electronic sound generator, which I personally find too noisy.

Bedtime is not the only time that the tinnitus sufferer might have issues with quiet backgrounds. Church settings, meetings, or sitting in a waiting room are also rather quiet locations, and in each you can expect that the patient's tinnitus is more pronounced to them. Therefore, plan ahead and perhaps incorporate some sort of distraction, such as using a cell phone to play music or some type of distracting sound or activity for the tinnitus patient. In this age of earbuds, it should be expected that the patient can achieve a relaxed state with minimal if any distraction to those around.

Denial

In most cases, those with long-term tinnitus probably have had some form of temporary tinnitus earlier in their life. That earlier version of tinnitus was probably associated with some loud event such as after a concert and probably lasted two or three days. Now, with a new round of tinnitus in their ear – and likely *not* associated with any prior loud event, the patient will probably be assuming that their tinnitus will go away soon and will not want to accept that they have chronic tinnitus.

I remember those days very well, waking up each morning to 'check' to see if I still had my tinnitus. And each morning, it was still there in my right ear, wailing away. Weeks of waiting for it to go away turned to months, and each day I remember thinking that there was no way I had the chronic form of tinnitus. It took months, really, for me to accept that this wasn't going away.

The issue that you will have regarding the patient's denial is that they may resist the need to get it checked out. "It'll go away soon enough" will be a phrase you can expect to hear. As you know, some forms of tinnitus have a true cause, whether it be buildup of ear wax or an acoustic neuroma. Medical attention is strongly suggested, and hopefully the patient will seek evaluation. But expect that in the initial phases of their tinnitus there will be a lack of motivation to get evaluated by a medical professional as the patient will in many cases be expecting the issue to go away on its own.

What you can do as a caregiver

Living with a tinnitus patient should cause no real change to your quality of life in the long term. Most of the issues listed above will be a factor in the initial months of tinnitus but will likely fade over time. Therefore, one of the best things that you can do when living with or providing care for a tinnitus sufferer is show *patience.* There will be good days and not so good days for *both of you.* Enjoying the good days and surviving the not so good days are key to maintaining a high quality of life for both of you.

Expect some disruption and adjustment to both your own life as well as that of the tinnitus sufferer. If hearing loss occurs with the tinnitus, there will be times that you will need to speak louder, or lean closer, while there will be other times that you can speak in a normal voice. Over time, you'll learn to recognize the environments that make hearing conversation hard for the patient (e.g. crowded rooms) in addition to those that have no effect. Try to avoid inadvertently pointing out the patient's tinnitus to others, such as might inadvertently occur if you ask a waiter to come closer because " . . . my husband can't hear you in here very well". Most tinnitus patients want to live as normal a life as possible, and any extraneous reminders of their tinnitus can add to their frustration.

Another thing to think about is to be able to separate the need to provide care from having to listen to whining (or being taken advantage of). There are times when the patient will have a genuine issue related to his or her tinnitus. There are other times when they are frustrated but having no real impediment resulting from their tinnitus. You are a support provider, not a verbal target. If there are times that you feel the patient is being unfair to you, let them know. In doing so, try to avoid verbal confrontation, as the patient may be having a particularly bad day or had some sort of trigger that you may not be aware of. Rather, try to guide the issue into a conversation, letting the patient know that their tone is not appropriate for the situation with you.

Some of the most difficult times as a tinnitus patient are when he or she is alone and inactive. Sitting alone in a room – especially a quiet one – can allow the mind to wander. And with tinnitus, there's a good chance that any thoughts are not particularly positive. Therefore, look to keep the tinnitus patient's mind active, and if possible, keep their body active as well. Outdoor walks or activity classes can be great for helping to distract from the annoyances of tinnitus.

Finally, learn as much as you can about tinnitus. Some patients themselves will dive into the research and treatment options. Others, such as those who may be in denial, will avoid any association with the condition and will in turn learn nothing about their condition. Be their 'behind the scenes' advocate by trying to learn as much as possible about tinnitus in order to help deflect any unnecessary triggers. In learning as much as you can as a caregiver, you can have quality discussions with the patient about treatment options and can discover ways to help improve the patient's quality of life such as through stress reduction, counseling, or even just through simple conversation with the patient.

In conclusion

Living with tinnitus is not easy. For some, living with a tinnitus sufferer is not easy, either. As we have discussed in this book, the most difficult times can be during the initial few months when the tinnitus can seem unbearable. Days, weeks, and months of waiting for the tinnitus to go away – only to find that no change ever occurs – can be frustrating to say the least, and can compound the patient's frustration. In providing support, you are not directly impacting their tinnitus, but you are indirectly helping improve the patient's quality of life. Stress, work, and certain social environments can make the tinnitus worse, and by limiting these stressors, there is a good chance that the tinnitus will seem less pronounced. Over time, as the patient learns coping mechanisms to deal with the tinnitus there will be a likely improvement in their self-reported level of tinnitus. As this occurs, you can expect to notice a general improvement in his or her quality of life.

Chapter 9: Preventing tinnitus

A S WE HAVE DISCUSSED in this book, tinnitus can range from a slightly detectable tone within the ear to a highly disruptive and debilitating condition. Particularly frustrating is that for the majority of people who develop tinnitus, there is no cure and as such the tinnitus will not likely diminish over time. Therefore, it is important for people who have not yet developed tinnitus to engage in behaviors that will reduce their likelihood of developing tinnitus. Whereas some types of tinnitus occur in response to non-preventable conditions such as acoustic neuromas, other forms of tinnitus are brought on by factors that are largely preventable, such as repeated exposure to loud music. Therefore, in this chapter we will look at some of the various influences that can increase an individual's chance for developing tinnitus as well as discuss some ways to help reduce tinnitus risk.

Probably because age-related hearing loss is such a prevalent factor in developing tinnitus, much of the research into preventing tinnitus is focused on youth including young children and adolescents. As we have discussed in an earlier chapter, children suffer from tinnitus at rates comparable to adults[136], but they complain less[38], which is thought to be due in part to the belief that the child feels that their tinnitus is normal[39].

Regardless of age, reducing the risk for developing tinnitus is an important concern given the healthcare costs associated with tinnitus care[137]. By increasing awareness of viable risk factors, the overall occurrence of tinnitus should be expected to decrease, in turn lowering the associated healthcare costs.

Risk factors for tinnitus

There have been a variety of risk factors reported for tinnitus, many of which have been discussed in earlier chapters of this book. Risk factors can further be separated into *definite* and *indefinite* risk factors[138]. Definite risk factors have been shown to cause tinnitus and include among other things repeated exposure to loud noise, head and neck trauma, diseases of the ear (e.g. otosclerosis), certain medications, or certain orthopedic diseases (e.g. temporomandibular joint syndrome). For example, noise exposure in children has been reported to increase the risk of developing tinnitus by 1.8 times[46].

Unfortunately, many of the risk factors associated with tinnitus are not truly preventable, such as developing certain diseases of the ear. Other conditions, such as exposure to loud noises are relatively preventable with a little effort. For example, noise barriers or the use of earplugs can significantly reduce the level of sound that reaches the ears and can in turn reduce long-term negative effects of the noise, thereby reducing the risk of developing tinnitus as a result of noise-associated hearing loss.

Indefinite risk factors have an association with tinnitus but are not known to have a consistent, direct cause. Examples of indirect risk factors include a family history of tinnitus, alcohol consumption, anxiety, depression, smoking, or overall poor health[138]. Like some of the "definite" risk factors, a few indefinite risk factors are preventable (e.g. smoking, alcohol consumption) while others such as a family history of tinnitus cannot be prevented. Furthermore, some factors can become complicated as the analysis becomes more involved. For example, while a family history of tinnitus increases one's risk for developing his or her own tinnitus, it has been reported that children are more likely to have tinnitus if their mother has it than their father[46].

Lifestyle aspects have also been shown to arise as risk factors for tinnitus. For example, lower income has been reported to increase the risk of developing tinnitus in young people[139]. Furthermore, reduced time sleeping has also been shown in children to increase tinnitus risk[46]. In such cases, lower income status has limited preventable aspects while increasing one's time asleep can be a factor that is more easily manipulated. However, a viable explanation as to how these risk factors actually result in the development of tinnitus remains to be determined.

Prevention tactics

At its simplest, the most effective way for a person to reduce his or her risk of developing tinnitus is to avoid those preventable situations that are associated with tinnitus. Avoiding loud music or sounds, getting enough sleep, and limiting exposure to smoking or alcohol can all be effective for reducing one's risk of developing tinnitus. Furthermore, given the association between hearing loss and tinnitus, it is worthwhile to focus on preventable factors that are known to influence hearing loss. For example, in addition to simply avoiding loud music, hearing loss risk can be reduced through the use of hearing protection, increasing the distance from the sound-generating source, or reducing the frequency of exposure to loud noise[140].

Other conditions associated with tinnitus such as family history are not as preventable. However, individuals with non-preventable risks should be able to help reduce their odds of developing tinnitus by ensuring that they receive scheduled hearing and/or medical checks and remain diligent in avoiding the many preventable triggers that are known to be associated with tinnitus. Similarly, for situations in which medication is needed for a particular medical condition, the patient might wish to discuss with his or her doctor their concerns regarding the medicine's risk for tinnitus and consider alternate medication options.

In addition to the individual person taking steps to reduce their risk for developing tinnitus, some countries have gone so far as to mandate noise level restrictions[140]. For example, the Netherlands conducts noise level assessments in restaurants and concert halls. If the noise is excessive, earplugs are made available along with the requirement that the noise level be reduced. While it remains to be determined as to the effectiveness of this plan – results could take decades to assess any change in overall rates of hearing loss or tinnitus – the premise seems worthwhile. However, enacting a similar mandate in the United States would take a significant amount of time and cost, and the basis for enacting such a plan in the United States would likely be dependent upon analyzing the effectiveness of the Netherlands' efforts.

Conclusion

Given that you have made it this far, I hope that this book has not only opened your eyes to the complexities involved in tinnitus, but also inspired and motivated you to continue to work to improve your quality of life. If you have tinnitus you are no doubt aware that it invades every aspect of your life. However, by utilizing some of the tactics and treatments outlined in this book, you can hopefully begin to suppress tinnitus to a level that allows you to forget that it's even there.

I wrote this book to help others who are suffering from tinnitus to understand that although tinnitus is quite common and seems at first to be a quite simple symptom, it is in fact a very complex event. So complex, in fact, that science still does not understand its range of involvement within the human body. Because of this involvement, tinnitus patients need to be aware of the level of effort it's going to take to get their tinnitus under control.

For anyone living with tinnitus, there has to be an acceptance that there is currently no cure. Any deviation from that can set oneself up to fall for false promises, scams, and an increased risk of being taken advantage of. Medicine is approaching a cure, but it's not looking to be happening in the immediate future. Therefore, we are left with treatments to help us deal with or reduce the effects of tinnitus. That in turn leads to the second aspect of tinnitus that sufferers must grasp – an understanding that it is going to take some effort to find the best treatment(s) for his or her tinnitus.

Successful treatment will likely take a concerted effort between you and your physician (or other healthcare provider), and may or may not include lifestyle changes, medications, and/or various psychological-oriented treatments to get you on track to living a relatively normal life free from the constraints of tinnitus. Despite medicine's progress in the search for a cure, we are not there yet; however, progress is ongoing and treatments have become more focused. It may just be a matter of time now before the cause – and the subsequent cure – of tinnitus is discovered. Given the tens of millions of people affected by tinnitus around the world, there is an incentive on many fronts to develop a viable treatment that leads to a cure. In the meantime, investigation into effective treatments are ongoing and a team effort between you and your healthcare provider can ensure that you are receiving the most effective treatments for your tinnitus.

Having lived for over 15 years with tinnitus that now exists in both ears, I can fully relate to what you are going through. I remember sitting through my own tinnitus evaluation hoping that I would have a quick fix for the high-pitched sound in my ear, only to find out soon after that no underlying cause could be found. That in turn woke me up to the realization of a life of constant ringing within my ears. So like you, I too have experienced the annoyance of not only the constant sound in your ears, but the anxiety associated with silent rooms, the frustration of family members asking me to turn down the television, and the struggle to understand conversation in a crowded room. But, through months of effort forcing myself to essentially ignore my own tinnitus, I have found that I no longer realize that it's there any more than I pay attention to the sound of a fan or other continuous noise in the background.

Because I found a way to basically ignore my own tinnitus, I wrote this book to help you also find a way to deal with yours. But rather than outlining a particular technique to you, my intent for this book was to provide you the basics and the background of tinnitus – what it is, how you can treat it, and how it can affect your quality of life. Most importantly, I wanted to provide you an overview of the most successful and recommended treatments so that you can have an honest conversation with your own healthcare provider in the event that your current tinnitus treatment is not working for you. This book was written with the intent of providing you the most up-to-date information, along with the sources of that information so that you can read more if you so choose.

After having read this book, I hope that you as a better-informed tinnitus patient have the motivation and drive to try to improve not only your own situation, but that of other tinnitus suffers as well. Read up on the recent research, promote effective treatment options, and encourage new suffers to get their medical evaluations. By improving your own life along with the lives of others, you can help reduce the impact of tinnitus and improve your quality of life along with the lives of other tinnitus sufferers.

I wish the best of luck to you and everyone involved.

Glossary

Acoustic neuroma: a benign tumor that grows on one of the nerves associated with the ear

Benign: not harmful

Benign paroxysmal positional vertigo: a condition of the inner ear thought to result from loose otoliths that can cause severe bouts of vertigo in response to certain head positions

Confounder: a factor in an experiment that can influence the results and must be accounted for

Cochlea: the organ of the inner ear shaped like a snail's shell which is responsible for receiving vibrations from the eardrum and converting them into electrical signals for transmission to the brain

Definite risk factor: a condition directly responsible for causing a condition or symptom

Dizziness: a sensation that results in the patient feeling as if he or she is spinning or moving while remaining stationary

Endolymph: the potassium-rich fluid contained within the membranous labyrinth of the ear

Equilibrium: a state of overall balance

Hair Cell: sensory receptors located within the auditory and vestibular organs of the ear that transmit a signal to the brain in response to detection of head movement or sound vibrations

Hypothesis: a prediction made based on available evidence

Indefinite risk factor: a condition that may play a role in developing or worsening a condition or symptom

Inner Ear: the portion of the ear within the temporal bone that contains the semicircular canals and cochlea

Labyrinth: the portion of the ear containing the hearing and balance organs

Ménière's Disease: a condition of the inner ear comprised of symptoms that include vertigo, tinnitus, hearing loss, and the sensation of ear fullness

Middle Ear: the central cavity of the inner ear comprised of the empty space within the temporal bone located inside of the eardrum

Nystagmus: involuntary eye movement

Objective tinnitus: tinnitus that is audible by another individual, such as might result from blood flow issues

Otolith: a small crystalline structure of the inner ear that plays a role in balance and equilibrium

Outer Ear: That portion of the ear that is visible, along with the auditory canal

Pinna: the external portion of the ear

Presbycusis: age-related hearing loss

Primary tinnitus: tinnitus that occurs without any known cause

Receptor: a small structure in the body that responds to a chemical message within the body

Secondary tinnitus: tinnitus that occurs in response to a recognized medical condition

Subjective tinnitus: tinnitus that is only detectable by the patient

Temporal bone: A bone that is positioned at the side and base of the skull which houses the vestibular and hearing organs

Vertigo: a sensation of spinning that is usually accompanied by a sudden loss of balance

Vestibular nerve: the eighth cranial nerve, responsible for transmitting hearing and sensory information from the inner ear to the brain

References

1.   Ekdale, E.G., *Form and function of the mammalian inner ear.* Journal of anatomy, 2016. **228**(2): p. 324-337.

2.   Gordon, C.R., et al., *Traumatic benign paroxysmal positional vertigo: diagnosis and treatment.* Harefuah, 2002. **141**(11): p. 944-7, 1012, 1011.

3.   Rask-Andersen, H., et al., *Human cochlea: anatomical characteristics and their relevance for cochlear implantation.* The Anatomical Record, 2012. **295**(11): p. 1791-1811.

4.   Hudspeth, A., *The hair cells of the inner ear.* Scientific American, 1983. **248**(1): p. 54-65.

5.   Viana, L.M., et al., *Cochlear neuropathy in human presbycusis: Confocal analysis of hidden hearing loss in post-mortem tissue.* Hearing research, 2015. **327**: p. 78-88.

6.   Purves, D., et al., *Neuroscience 2nd Edition. Sunderland (MA) Sinauer Associates.* 2001, Inc.

7.   Stephens, S., *The treatment of tinnitus — a historical perspective.* The Journal of Laryngology & Otology, 1984. **98**(10): p. 963-972.

8.   Vernon, J., *The history of masking as applied to tinnitus.* The Journal of laryngology and otology. Supplement, 1981(4): p. 76-79.

9.   Celsus, A.C. and W.G. Spencer, *De medicina. With an English translation by WG Spencer.* 1935:

London; Harvard University Press: Cambridge, Mass.

10. Swain, S.K., et al., *Tinnitus and its current treatment–Still an enigma in medicine.* Journal of the Formosan Medical Association, 2016. **115**(3): p. 139-144.

11. Langguth, B., et al., *Tinnitus: causes and clinical management.* The Lancet Neurology, 2013. **12**(9): p. 920-930.

12. Tunkel, D.E., et al., *Clinical practice guideline: tinnitus.* Otolaryngology–Head and Neck Surgery, 2014. **151**(2_suppl): p. S1-S40.

13. Lockwood, A.H., *Tinnitus.* Neurologic clinics, 2005. **23**(3): p. 893-900.

14. Elgoyhen, A.B., et al., *Tinnitus: perspectives from human neuroimaging.* Nature Reviews Neuroscience, 2015. **16**(10): p. 632.

15. Henry, J.A., K.C. Dennis, and M.A. Schechter, *General review of tinnitus: prevalence, mechanisms, effects, and management.* Journal of speech, language, and hearing research, 2005. **48**(5): p. 1204-1235.

16. Møller, A.R., *Tinnitus: presence and future.* Progress in brain research, 2007. **166**: p. 3-16.

17. Yankaskas, K., *Prelude: noise-induced tinnitus and hearing loss in the military.* Hearing research, 2013. **295**: p. 3-8.

18.   Hinton, D.E., et al., *Tinnitus among Cambodian refugees: relationship to PTSD severity.* Journal of traumatic stress, 2006. **19**(4): p. 541-546.

19.   McKENNA, L., R.S. HALLAM, and R. HINCHCLIFFEf, *The prevalence of psychological disturbance in neuro-otology outpatients.* Clinical Otolaryngology, 1991. **16**(5): p. 452-456.

20.   Saldanha, A.D.D., et al., *Are temporomandibular disorders and tinnitus associated?* CRANIO®, 2012. **30**(3): p. 166-171.

21.   Lee, S.H., et al., *Otologic manifestations of acoustic neuroma.* Acta oto-laryngologica, 2015. **135**(2): p. 140-146.

22.   Lindblad, A.-C., B. Hagerman, and U. Rosenhall, *Noise-induced tinnitus: a comparison between four clinical groups without apparent hearing loss.* Noise and Health, 2011. **13**(55): p. 423.

23.   Baguley, D., et al., *Tinnitus: A Multidisciplinary Approach. Chichester.* 2013, Wiley-Blackwell.

24.   Atik, A., *Pathophysiology and treatment of tinnitus: an elusive disease.* Indian Journal of Otolaryngology and Head & Neck Surgery, 2014. **66**(1): p. 1-5.

25.   Tang, J., B. Ji, and L. Liu, *Study of hearing loss in 200 patients with subjective tinnitus.* Lin chuang er bi yan hou tou jing wai ke za zhi= Journal of clinical otorhinolaryngology, head, and neck surgery, 2011. **25**(16): p. 726-729.

26.   Davis, A. and E.A. Rafaie, *Epidemiology of tinnitus.* Tinnitus handbook, 2000: p. 1-23.

27.   Norena, A., et al., *Psychoacoustic characterization of the tinnitus spectrum: implications for the underlying mechanisms of tinnitus.* Audiology and Neurotology, 2002. **7**(6): p. 358-369.

28.   House, J.W. and D. Brackman. *Tinnitus: surgical treatment.* in *Ciba foundation symposium.* 1981.

29.   Jackson, P., *A comparison of the effects of eighth nerve section with lidocaine on tinnitus.* The Journal of Laryngology & Otology, 1985. **99**(7): p. 663-666.

30.   Mühlnickel, W., et al., *Reorganization of auditory cortex in tinnitus.* Proceedings of the National Academy of Sciences, 1998. **95**(17): p. 10340-10343.

31.   Shargorodsky, J., G.C. Curhan, and W.R. Farwell, *Prevalence and characteristics of tinnitus among US adults.* The American journal of medicine, 2010. **123**(8): p. 711-718.

32.   Heller, A.J., *Classification and epidemiology of tinnitus.* Otolaryngologic Clinics of North America, 2003. **36**(2): p. 239-248.

33.   Pinto, P.C.L., T.G. Sanchez, and S. Tomita, *The impact of gender, age and hearing loss on tinnitus severity.* Brazilian journal of otorhinolaryngology, 2010. **76**(1): p. 18-24.

34.   Hiller, W. and G. Goebel, *Factors influencing tinnitus loudness and annoyance.* Archives of

142

Otolaryngology–Head & Neck Surgery, 2006. **132**(12): p. 1323-1330.

35. Baguley, D.M. and D. McFerran, *Tinnitus in childhood.* International journal of pediatric otorhinolaryngology, 1999. **49**(2): p. 99-105.

36. Niskar, A.S., et al., *Estimated prevalence of noise-induced hearing threshold shifts among children 6 to 19 years of age: the Third National Health and Nutrition Examination Survey, 1988–1994, United States.* Pediatrics, 2001. **108**(1): p. 40-43.

37. Vogel, I., et al., *Adolescents risky MP3-player listening and its psychosocial correlates.* Health education research, 2011. **26**(2): p. 254-264.

38. Savastano, M., G. Marioni, and C. de Filippis, *Tinnitus in children without hearing impairment.* International journal of pediatric otorhinolaryngology, 2009. **73**: p. S13-S15.

39. Shetye, A. and V. Kennedy, *Tinnitus in children: an uncommon symptom?* Archives of disease in childhood, 2010. **95**(8): p. 645-648.

40. Mills, R., D. Albert, and C. Brain, *Tinnitus in childhood.* Clinical Otolaryngology, 1986. **11**(6): p. 431-434.

41. Leensen, M.C., J.A. de Laat, and W.A. Dreschler, *Speech-in-noise screening tests by internet, part 1: test evaluation for noise-induced hearing loss identification.* International journal of audiology, 2011. **50**(11): p. 823-834.

42. de Lourdes Quintanilla-Dieck, M., M.A. Artunduaga, and R.D. Eavey, *Intentional exposure to loud music: the second MTV. com survey reveals an opportunity to educate.* The Journal of pediatrics, 2009. **155**(4): p. 550-555. e5.

43. Hoffman, H.J. and G.W. Reed, *Epidemiology of tinnitus.* Tinnitus: Theory and management, 2004: p. 16-41.

44. Krog, N.H., B. Engdahl, and K. Tambs, *The association between tinnitus and mental health in a general population sample: Results from the HUNT Study.* Journal of Psychosomatic Research, 2010. **69**(3): p. 289-298.

45. Mahboubi, H., et al., *The prevalence and characteristics of tinnitus in the youth population of the United States.* The Laryngoscope, 2013. **123**(8): p. 2001-2008.

46. Park, B., et al., *Analysis of the Prevalence of and Risk Factors for Tinnitus in a Young Population.* Otology & Neurotology, 2014. **35**(7): p. 1218-1222.

47. Lewis, R.C., R.R. Gershon, and R.L. Neitzel, *Estimation of permanent noise-induced hearing loss in an urban setting.* Environmental science & technology, 2013. **47**(12): p. 6393-6399.

48. Nondahl, D.M., et al., *The ten-year incidence of tinnitus among older adults.* International Journal of Audiology, 2010. **49**(8): p. 580-585.

49.   Stouffer, J., et al., *Tinnitus as a function of duration and etiology: counselling implications*. The American Journal of Otology, 1991. **12**(3): p. 188-194.

50.   Gopinath, B., et al., *Incidence, Persistence, and Progression of Tinnitus Symptoms in Older Adults: The Blue Mountains Hearing Study*. Ear and Hearing, 2010. **31**(3): p. 407-412.

51.   Hallam, R., S. Rachman, and R. Hinchcliffe, *Psychological aspects of tinnitus*. Vol. 3. 1984. 31-53.

52.   Hazell, J., *Management of tinnitus*, in *Diseases of the ear*, H. Ludman and T. Wright, Editors. 1998. p. 202–215.

53.   Roland, P.S., et al., *Clinical practice guideline: Cerumen impaction*. Otolaryngology–Head and Neck Surgery, 2008. **139**(3_suppl_1): p. S1-S21.

54.   Noell, C. and W. Meyerhoff, *Tinnitus. Diagnosis and treatment of this elusive symptom*. Geriatrics, 2003. **58**(2): p. 28-34.

55.   Vernon, J., R. Johnson, and A. Schleuning, *The characteristics and natural history of tinnitus in Meniere's disease*. Otolaryngologic Clinics of North America, 1980. **13**(4): p. 611-619.

56.   El-Shunnar Suliman, K., et al., *Primary care for tinnitus: practice and opinion among GPs in England*. Journal of Evaluation in Clinical Practice, 2011. **17**(4): p. 684-692.

57. Møller, A.R., *Pathophysiology of tinnitus.* Otolaryngologic Clinics of North America, 2003. **36**(2): p. 249-266.

58. Melding, P.S., R.J. Goodey, and P.R. Thorne, *The use of intravenous lignocaine in the diagnosis and treatment of tinnitus.* The Journal of Laryngology & Otology, 2007. **92**(2): p. 115-121.

59. Trellakis, S., J. Lautermann, and G. Lehnerdt, *Lidocaine: neurobiological targets and effects on the auditory system,* in *Progress in Brain Research,* B. Langguth, et al., Editors. 2007, Elsevier. p. 303-322.

60. Beebe Palumbo, D., et al., *The Management and Outcomes of Pharmacological Treatments for Tinnitus.* Current Neuropharmacology, 2015. **13**(5): p. 692-700.

61. Sönmez, O., et al., *The evaluation of ozone and betahistine in the treatment of tinnitus.* European Archives of Oto-Rhino-Laryngology, 2013. **270**(7): p. 1999-2006.

62. Podoshin, L., M. Fradis, and Y.B. David, *Treatment of tinnitus by intratympanic instillation of lignocaine (lidocaine) 2 per cent through ventilation tubes.* The Journal of Laryngology & Otology, 2007. **106**(7): p. 603-606.

63. Podoshin, L., et al., *Idiopathic Subjective Tinnitus Treated by Amitriptyline Hydrochloride/Biofeedback.* The international tinnitus journal, 1995. **1**(1): p. 54-60.

64.   Sullivan, M., et al., *A randomized trial of nortriptyline for severe chronic tinnitus: Effects on depression, disability, and tinnitus symptoms.* Archives of Internal Medicine, 1993. **153**(19): p. 2251-2259.

65.   Mendis, D. and M. Johnston, *An unusual case of prolonged tinnitus following low-dose amitriptyline.* Journal of Psychopharmacology, 2008. **22**(5): p. 574-575.

66.   Johnson, R.M., R. Brummett, and A. Schleuning, *Use of alprazolam for relief of tinnitus: A double-blind study.* Archives of Otolaryngology–Head & Neck Surgery, 1993. **119**(8): p. 842-845.

67.   Jalali, M.M., et al., *The effects of alprazolam on tinnitus: a cross-over randomized clinical trial.* Medical Science Monitor, 2009. **15**(11): p. 155-160.

68.   Han, S.-S., et al., *Clonazepam Quiets tinnitus: a randomised crossover study with <em>Ginkgo Biloba</em&gt.* Journal of Neurology, Neurosurgery & Psychiatry, 2012. **83**(8): p. 821.

69.   Bauer, C.A. and T.J. Brozoski, *Effect of Gabapentin on the sensation and impact of tinnitus.* The Laryngoscope, 209. **116**(5): p. 675-681.

70.   Witsell, D.L., et al., *Treatment of Tinnitus With Gabapentin: A Pilot Study.* Otology & Neurotology, 2007. **28**(1): p. 11-15.

71. Dobie, R.A., *A review of randomized clinical trials in tinnitus.* The Laryngoscope, 1999. **109**(8): p. 1202-1211.

72. Berkiten, G., et al., *Vitamin B12 levels in patients with tinnitus and effectiveness of vitamin B12 treatment on hearing threshold and tinnitus.* B-ENT, 2013. **9**: p. 111-116.

73. Coelho, C., et al., *Zinc to Treat Tinnitus in the Elderly: A Randomized Placebo Controlled Crossover Trial.* Otology & Neurotology, 2013. **34**(6): p. 1146-1154.

74. Ernst, E. and C. Stevinson, *Ginkgo biloba for tinnitus: a review.* Clinical Otolaryngology & Allied Sciences, 1999. **24**(3): p. 164-167.

75. Vernon, J. and A. Schleuning, *Tinnitus: A New Management.* The Laryngoscope, 1978. **88**(3): p. 413-419.

76. Coles, R.R.A., J.L. Baskill, and J.B. Sheldrake, *Measurement and management of tinnitus Part II. Management.* The Journal of Laryngology & Otology, 2007. **99**(1): p. 1-10.

77. Henry, J.A., et al., *Using Therapeutic Sound With Progressive Audiologic Tinnitus Management.* Trends in Amplification, 2008. **12**(3): p. 188-209.

78. Norena, A., C. Micheyl, and S. Chery-Croze, *An auditory negative after-image as a human model of tinnitus.* Hearing Research, 2000. **149**(1): p. 24-32.

79. Okamoto, H., et al., *Listening to tailor-made notched music reduces tinnitus loudness and*

tinnitus-related auditory cortex activity. Proceedings of the National Academy of Sciences, 2010. **107**(3): p. 1207.

80.   Hobson, J., E. Chisholm, and A. El Refaie, *Sound therapy (masking) in the management of tinnitus in adults.* Cochrane Database of Systematic Reviews, 2012(11).

81.   Kaldo, V., et al., *Use of a self-help book with weekly therapist contact to reduce tinnitus distress: A randomized controlled trial.* Journal of Psychosomatic Research, 2007. **63**(2): p. 195-202.

82.   Cima, R.F.F., et al., *Specialised treatment based on cognitive behaviour therapy versus usual care for tinnitus: a randomised controlled trial.* The Lancet, 2012. **379**(9830): p. 1951-1959.

83.   Martinez-Devesa, P., et al., *Cognitive behavioural therapy for tinnitus.* Cochrane Database of Systematic Reviews, 2010(9).

84.   Andersson, G. and L. Lyttkens, *A meta-analytic review of psychological treatments for tinnitus.* British Journal of Audiology, 1999. **33**(4): p. 201-210.

85.   Jastreboff, P.J., et al., *Phantom auditory sensation in rats: An animal model for tinnitus.* Behavioral Neuroscience, 1988. **102**(6): p. 811-822.

86.   Tan, K.-Q., et al., *Comparative study on therapeutic effects of acupuncture, Chinese herbs and Western medicine on nervous tinnitus.* Zhongguo zhen jiu =

Chinese acupuncture & moxibustion, 2007. **27**(4): p. 249-251.

87. Kim, J.-I., et al., *Acupuncture for the treatment of tinnitus: a systematic review of randomized clinical trials.* BMC Complementary and Alternative Medicine, 2012. **12**(1): p. 97.

88. Habesoglu, M., et al., *Is there any predictor for tinnitus outcome in different types of otologic surgery?* European Archives of Oto-Rhino-Laryngology, 2013. **270**(8): p. 2225-2229.

89. Baba, S., T. Yagi, and T. Fujikura, *Subjective Evaluation and Overall Satisfaction after Tympanoplasty for Chronic Simple Suppurative Otitis Media.* Journal of Nippon Medical School, 2004. **71**(1): p. 17-24.

90. Moody-Antonio, S. and J.W. House, *Hearing Outcome After Concurrent Endolymphatic Shunt and Vestibular Nerve Section.* Otology & Neurotology, 2003. **24**(3): p. 453-459.

91. BROWNING, G.G. and S. GATEHOUSE, *The prevalence of middle ear disease in the adult British population.* Clinical Otolaryngology & Allied Sciences, 1992. **17**(4): p. 317-321.

92. Sobrinho, P., C. Oliveira, and A. Venosa, *Long-term follow-up of tinnitus in patients with otosclerosis after stapes surgery.* International Tinnitus Journal, 2004. **10**(2): p. 197-201.

93.   Sismanis, A. and W.R.K. Smoker, *Pulsatile tinnitus: Recent advances in diagnosis.* The Laryngoscope, 1994. **104**(6): p. 681-688.

94.   Gersdorff, M., et al., *Tinnitus and otosclerosis.* European Archives of Oto-Rhino-Laryngology, 2000. **257**(6): p. 314-316.

95.   Ayache, D., F. Earally, and P. Elbaz, *Characteristics and Postoperative Course of Tinnitus in Otosclerosis.* Otology & Neurotology, 2003. **24**(1): p. 48-51.

96.   Figueiredo, R.R., A.A. de Azevedo, and N. de Oliveira Penido, *Ménière's Disease and Tinnitus*, in *Up to Date on Meniere's Disease*. 2017, InTech.

97.   Minor, L.B., D.A. Schessel, and J.P. Carey, *Meniere's disease.* Current opinion in neurology, 2004. **17**(1): p. 9-16.

98.   Ishiyama, G., I. Lopez, and A. Ishiyama, *Aquaporins and Meniere's disease.* Current Opinion in Otolaryngology & Head and Neck Surgery, 2006. **14**(5): p. 332-336.

99.   Rauch, S.D., *Clinical Hints and Precipitating Factors in Patients Suffering from Meniere's Disease.* Otolaryngologic Clinics of North America, 2010. **43**(5): p. 1011-1017.

100.   Kangasniemi, E. and E. Hietikko, *The theory of autoimmunity in Meniere's disease is lacking evidence.* Auris Nasus Larynx, 2018. **45**(3): p. 399-406.

101.   Vrabec, J.T., *Herpes simplex virus and Meniere's Disease.* The Laryngoscope, 2003. **113**(9): p. 1431-1438.

102.   Bjorne, A., A. Berven, and G. Agerberg, *Cervical Signs and Symptoms in Patients with Meniere's Disease: A Controlled Study.* CRANIO®, 1998. **16**(3): p. 194-202.

103.   Söderman, A.C.H., et al., *Stress as a Trigger of Attacks in Menière's Disease. A Case-Crossover Study.* The Laryngoscope, 2004. **114**(10): p. 1843-1848.

104.   Brookes, G.B., A.R. Maw, and M.J. Coleman, *'Costen's syndrome'—correlation or coincidence: a review of 45 patients with temporomandibular joint dysfunction, otalgia and other aural symptoms.* Clinical Otolaryngology & Allied Sciences, 1980. **5**(1): p. 23-36.

105.   Lee, C.-F., et al., *Increased risk of tinnitus in patients with temporomandibular disorder: a retrospective population-based cohort study.* European Archives of Oto-Rhino-Laryngology, 2016. **273**(1): p. 203-208.

106.   Morgan, D.H., *Tinnitus of TMJ Origin: A Preliminary Report.* CRANIO®, 1992. **10**(2): p. 124-129.

107.   Campbell, K., *Tinnitus and vertigo.* Archives of Otolaryngology–Head & Neck Surgery, 1993. **119**(4): p. 474-474.

108. Nikolopoulos, T.P., et al., *Acoustic Neuroma Growth: A Systematic Review of the Evidence.* Otology & Neurotology, 2010. **31**(3): p. 478-485.

109. McLaughlin, E.J., et al., *Quality of Life in Acoustic Neuroma Patients.* Otology & Neurotology, 2015. **36**(4): p. 653-656.

110. Moffat, D.A., et al., *Clinical acumen and vestibular schwannoma.* The American journal of otology, 1998. **19**(1): p. 82-87.

111. Eggermont, J.J., *On the pathophysiology of tinnitus; A review and a peripheral model.* Hearing Research, 1990. **48**(1): p. 111-123.

112. Baguley, D.M., et al., *The Clinical Characteristics of Tinnitus in Patients with Vestibular Schwannoma.* Skull Base, 2006. **16**(2): p. 49-58.

113. Dietrich, V., et al., *Cortical reorganization in patients with high frequency cochlear hearing loss.* Hearing Research, 2001. **158**(1): p. 95-101.

114. McClelland, S.I., et al., *Impact of Race and Insurance Status on Surgical Approach for Cervical Spondylotic Myelopathy in the United States: A Population-Based Analysis.* Spine, 2017. **42**(3): p. 186-194.

115. Fusco, M.R., et al., *Current practices in vestibular schwannoma management: A survey of American and Canadian neurosurgeons.* Clinical Neurology and Neurosurgery, 2014. **127**: p. 143-148.

116. Negrila-Mezei, A., R. Enache, and C. Sarafoleanu, *Tinnitus in elderly population: clinic*

153

correlations and impact upon QoL. Journal of Medicine and Life, 2011. **4**(4): p. 412-416.

117. Lasisi, A.O. and O. Gureje, *Prevalence of Insomnia and Impact on Quality of Life among Community Elderly Subjects with Tinnitus.* Annals of Otology, Rhinology & Laryngology, 2011. **120**(4): p. 226-230.

118. Tyler, R.S., S.A. Gogel, and A.K. Gehringer, *Tinnitus activities treatment*, in *Progress in Brain Research*, B. Langguth, et al., Editors. 2007, Elsevier. p. 425-434.

119. Sahley, T.L. and R.H. Nodar, *A biochemical model of peripheral tinnitus11Portions of this article were presented at The Dartmouth-Hitchcock Medical Center Conference on Tinnitus: New Perspectives on Diagnosis and Management, Lebanon, NH, 13–14 August 1999.* Hearing Research, 2001. **152**(1): p. 43-54.

120. Cima, R.F.F., G. Crombez, and J.W.S. Vlaeyen, *Catastrophizing and Fear of Tinnitus Predict Quality of Life in Patients With Chronic Tinnitus.* Ear and Hearing, 2011. **32**(5): p. 634-641.

121. Harrop-Griffiths, J., et al., *Chronic tinnitus: Association with psychiatric diagnoses.* Journal of Psychosomatic Research, 1987. **31**(5): p. 613-621.

122. Zöger, S., J. Svedlund, and K.-M. Holgers, *Relationship Between Tinnitus Severity and Psychiatric Disorders.* Psychosomatics, 2006. **47**(4): p. 282-288.

154

123. Geocze, L., et al., *Systematic review on the evidences of an association between tinnitus and depression.* Brazilian Journal of Otorhinolaryngology, 2013. **79**(1): p. 106-111.

124. Bartels, H., et al., *The Impact of Type D Personality on Health-Related Quality of Life in Tinnitus Patients Is Mainly Mediated by Anxiety and Depression.* Otology & Neurotology, 2010. **31**(1): p. 11-18.

125. Mols, F. and J. Denollet, *Type D personality in the general population: a systematic review of health status, mechanisms of disease, and work-related problems.* Health and Quality of Life Outcomes, 2010. **8**(1): p. 9.

126. Tyler, R.S. and L.J. Baker, *Difficulties Experienced by Tinnitus Sufferers.* Journal of Speech and Hearing Disorders, 1983. **48**(2): p. 150-154.

127. Durai, M., M.G. O'Keeffe, and G.D. Searchfield, *The Personality Profile of Tinnitus Sufferers and a Nontinnitus Control Group.* Journal of the American Academy of Audiology, 2017. **28**(4): p. 271-282.

128. Zeman, F., et al., *Which tinnitus-related aspects are relevant for quality of life and depression: results from a large international multicentre sample.* Health and Quality of Life Outcomes, 2014. **12**(1): p. 7.

129. Carpenter-Thompson, J.R., E. McAuley, and F.T. Husain, *Physical Activity, Tinnitus Severity, and*

Improved Quality of Life. Ear and Hearing, 2015. **36**(5): p. 574-581.

130. Davis, A.C., *Hearing Disorders in the Population: First Phase Findings of the MRC National Study of Hearing*, in *Hearing Science and Hearing Disorders*. 1983, Academic Press: London. p. 35-60.

131. Holgers, K.M., S. Zöger, and K. Svedlund, *Predictive factors for development of severe tinnitus suffering-further characterisation.* International Journal of Audiology, 2005. **44**(10): p. 584-592.

132. Lockwood, A.H., R.J. Salvi, and R.F. Burkard, *Tinnitus.* New England Journal of Medicine, 2002. **347**(12): p. 904-910.

133. Alhazmi, F., et al., *An Investigation of the Impact of Tinnitus Perception on the Quality of Life.* Journal of Phonetics and Audiology, 2016. **2**(1).

134. Riedl, D., et al., *The influence of tinnitus acceptance on the quality of life and psychological distress in patients with chronic tinnitus.* Noise & Health, 2015. **17**(78): p. 374-381.

135. Nondahl, D.M., et al., *The Impact of Tinnitus on Quality of Life in Older Adults.* Journal of the American Academy of Audiology, 2007. **18**(3): p. 257-266.

136. Baguley, D.M. and D.J. McFerran, *Tinnitus in childhood.* International Journal of Pediatric Otorhinolaryngology, 1999. **49**(2): p. 99-105.

137. Stockdale, D., et al., *An economic evaluation of the healthcare cost of tinnitus management in the UK.*

BMC Health Services Research, 2017. **17**(1): p. 577.

138. Çelik, O., *Risk factors for tinnitus.* Journal of International Advanced Otology, 2015. **11**.

139. Brunnberg, E., M. Lindén-Boström, and M. Berglund, *Tinnitus and hearing loss in 15–16-year-old students: Mental health symptoms, substance use, and exposure in school.* International Journal of Audiology, 2008. **47**(11): p. 688-694.

140. de Laat, J.A.P.M., L. van Deelen, and K. Wiefferink, *Hearing Screening and Prevention of Hearing Loss in Adolescents.* Journal of Adolescent Health, 2016. **59**(3): p. 243-245.

Other published books written by Mark Knoblauch

In addition to *Outlining Tinnitus*, Mark has released two prior books as part of his *Labyrinth* series and has published one book designed to assist everyday writers in the process of writing and publishing their own book.

Mark is also working on several books focused on diet as well as exercise, and if you are interested in academic writing, be sure to watch for the release of his upcoming edited book detailing how to improve your professional writing skills.

Overcoming Ménière's. How changing your lifestyle can change your life.

ISBN# 978-1-7320674-7-9.

Overcoming Ménière's provides the reader a detailed overview of Ménière's including the involved anatomy as well as the most recent research. By detailing his own Ménière's journey as well as what has worked for his own battle with Ménière's, Mark intends to provide other Ménière's sufferers a pathway which they themselves can following in order to find similar relief from the devastating effects of Ménière's disease.

Understanding BPPV. Outlining the causes and effects of Benign Paroxysmal Positional Vertigo

ISBN# 978-1-7320674-1-7

Benign Paroxysmal Positional Vertigo is a condition that triggers vertigo when the head is placed in a particular position. Furthermore, the vertigo ceases once the head is repositioned. Despite the somewhat forceful symptoms inherent to BPPV, the underlying cause of BPPV is relatively minor and can typically be fixed with a simple visit to a medical professional's office.

Because of his own experience with BPPV, Mark wrote *Understanding BPPV* so that everyone affected by this condition can have a solid resource guide outlining just what BPPV is, how it occurs, and how it is treated. Particular attention is focused on the anatomy of the ear, and how this anatomy is involved in generating the symptoms associated with BPPV. Mark also details the latest research into BPPV and provides an overview of the various diagnostic tests and treatments used to help BPPV patients in many cases get back to a vertigo-free life.

Essentials of Writing and Publishing your Self-Help Book

ISBN# 978-1-7320674-9-3

Some people elect to transform their own experiences and successes into a self-help book that outlines how they persevered through their difficult times. As a potential self-help book author yourself, you might be struggling to get started, get finished, or just need tips on how to finally get your advice and ideas onto bookstore shelves. *Essentials of Writing and Publishing Your Self-Help Book* is filled with information that will help walk you through the process of producing a quality self-help book. You'll be exposed to strategies that will help get you through the various stages of book production, gain insight into the options you have available for publication of your book, and review the individual steps and requirements necessary to get your advice from paper to a finished book.

Hidden down deep inside of us, we all have a book waiting to be written. The tips and techniques outlined in this book are designed to help you bring your ideas, successes, and lessons to life in the form of your own self-help book.

Let others know!

If you found this or any of Mark's other books informative, *please take the time and post a review online*! Reviews help get exposure for the books and thereby improve the chances that others will be able to benefit from the material as well!

Image Credits

Cover Image: rudall30/shutterstock.com

Image 1.1 MedicalArtInc/shutterstock.com
Image 1.2 Maxcreatnz/shutterstock.com
Image 1.3 Alexilusmedical/shutterstock.com

Made in the USA
Monee, IL
16 March 2023

29982541R00095